Praise for *A Nurse's Step-By-Step Guide to Transitioning to the Professional Nurse Role*

"Excellently … es
they may fac… …
challenges ar… …very
nurse could … …
looking to in… …

…CHPN
…ifornia
…Center

"Thomas, M… …
perspective t… …
consummate … …

…less Jr.
…tialing
…arning
…n.com

"*A Nurse's Ste…* …se
Role is a trem… …
nursing, stud… …ly
be advising p… …ant
topics in a wa… …
This book is … …
professional r… …

…), RN
…ration
…ersity

"*A Nurse's Step-By-Step G…… to Transitioning to the Professional Nurse Role* is an easy-to-read and very informative book for the student or new graduate nurse. The authors have provided a straightforward narrative that covers all the information needed to begin the transition from student to registered professional nurse. This is a must-read for new grads!"

–Mimi Haskins, DNP, RN, CNS, CMSRN
Corporate Nurse Educator, Catholic Health

"*A Nurse's Step-By-Step Guide to Transitioning to the Professional Nurse Role* is comprehensive, reliable, and impeccably researched. Readers will learn the expectations and essential behaviors for specific, measurable outcomes. The 10 chapters cover the core concepts of professionalism in a healthcare framework and provide specific strategies to cope with and reduce stress, take the NCLEX, deal with legal and ethical issues, and navigate leadership. It should be a textbook for every school of nursing to give students a perspective of what is to come and prepare them for transitioning into practice. The book also guides clinical preceptors and managers in providing quality orientation, support, and assistance—and in developing key strategies for retaining newly licensed nurses."

–Hazel W. Chappell, MSN, RN
Director, Nursing Continuing Education
University of Kentucky

A NURSE'S STEP-BY-STEP GUIDE TO
TRANSITIONING TO THE PROFESSIONAL NURSE ROLE

CYNTHIA M. THOMAS, EDD, MS, RNC
CONSTANCE E. MCINTOSH, EDD, MBA, RN
JENNIFER S. MENSIK, PHD, MBA, RN, NEA-BC, FAAN

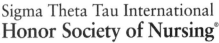

Sigma Theta Tau International
Honor Society of Nursing®

Copyright © 2016 by Sigma Theta Tau International

The Honor Society of Nursing, Sigma Theta Tau International (STTI) is a nonprofit organization founded in 1922 whose mission is to support the learning, knowledge, and professional development of nurses committed to making a difference in health worldwide. Members include practicing nurses, instructors, researchers, policymakers, entrepreneurs and others. STTI's 499 chapters are located at 698 institutions of higher education throughout Australia, Botswana, Brazil, Canada, Colombia, Ghana, Hong Kong, Japan, Kenya, Malawi, Mexico, the Netherlands, Pakistan, Portugal, Singapore, South Africa, South Korea, Swaziland, Sweden, Taiwan, Tanzania, United Kingdom, United States, and Wales. More information about STTI can be found online at www.nursingsociety.org.

Sigma Theta Tau International
550 West North Street
Indianapolis, IN, USA 46202

To order additional books, buy in bulk, or order for corporate use, contact Nursing Knowledge International at 888.NKI.4YOU (888.654.4968/US and Canada) or +1.317.634.8171 (outside US and Canada).

To request a review copy for course adoption, e-mail solutions@nursingknowledge.org or call 888.NKI.4YOU (888.654.4968/US and Canada) or +1.317.634.8171 (outside US and Canada).

To request author information, or for speaker or other media requests, contact Marketing, Honor Society of Nursing, Sigma Theta Tau International at 888.634.7575 (US and Canada) or +1.317.634.8171 (outside US and Canada).

ISBN: 9781940446226
EPUB ISBN: 9781940446233
PDF ISBN: 9781940446240
MOBI ISBN: 9781940446257

Library of Congress Cataloging-in-Publication Data

Thomas, Cynthia M., 1951- , author.
A nurse's step-by-step guide to transitioning to the professional nurse role / Cynthia M. Thomas, Constance E. McIntosh, Jennifer S. Mensik.
  p. ; cm.
Includes bibliographical references.
ISBN 978-1-940446-22-6 (alk. paper) -- ISBN 978-1-940446-23-3 (epub) -- ISBN 978-1-940446-24-0 (pdf) -- ISBN 978-1-940446-25-7 (mobi)
I. McIntosh, Constance E., 1967- , author. II. Mensik, Jennifer, author. III. Sigma Theta Tau International, publisher. IV. Title.
[DNLM: 1. Nurses--United States. 2. Education, Nursing--United States. 3. Nurse's Role--United States. 4. Vocational Guidance--United States. WY 16 AA1]
RT82
610.7306'9--dc23
                              2015033510

First Printing, 2015

Publisher: Dustin Sullivan
Acquisitions Editor: Emily Hatch
Editorial Coordinator: Paula Jeffers
Cover Designer: Rebecca Batchelor
Interior Design/Page Layout: Rebecca Batchelor
Cover and Text Illustrations: Megan Johns

Principal Book Editor: Carla Hall
Development and Project Editor: Kevin Kent
Copy Editor: Rebecca Whitney
Proofreader: Todd Lothery
Indexer: Jane Palmer

Dedication

To my husband, John, who has provided the support and
encouragement to push forward.
–Cindy

For my dad, the late James Edwin Ross, and my mom,
the late Marilyn Louise Ross.
–Connie

For Evan and Ethan, who want to know if I am writing
another book, as they know their bedtime tends to get
pushed back a little when I am.
–Jennifer

Acknowledgments

Nurses never really work alone, and this book would not have been possible without the help and encouragement of others. I would like to thank Connie McIntosh and Jennifer Mensik, for their enthusiasm and contributions to this book. Their willingness to give up nights and weekends to write and rewrite the contents of this book are much appreciated. I would also like to thank Marilyn Ryan, for believing in me and for serving patiently as a wonderful mentor. Without her encouragement and persistence, I may not be where I am today. A huge thanks to the many students and nurses whom I have been privileged to work alongside, to start their careers or to provide direction and a push to continue their education.

Lastly, I want to thank my husband, John, for his technical support and encouragement to try new things. Thank you to my children and grandchildren: my daughter Brandi and her husband Marcus; my son Jesse and his wife Jennifer; and my grandchildren Zoe, Max, and Cooper. Of course, many thanks must go to Mimi, our Westie, who tirelessly sat by my side as I worked and insisted that I take regular breaks by taking her outdoors or getting a little something to eat.

–Cindy

With gratefulness, I thank Cindy Thomas, for her encouragement of me and for her unconditional belief in this project. Thank you to Jennifer Mensik, for her enthusiasm and positive work ethic. Cindy and Jennifer are truly incredible professionals.

With sincerity, a hearty thank-you to my husband, David, and our children Gavan, Claire, and Ross. For many months, my nights and weekends were spent writing this book, and I so appreciated my family's support. On a daily basis, David provides me with encouragement and love, and because of it, I am blessed.

A special thank-you to my aunt, Patricia Yeager, who dedicated her life to nursing. You are a great source of inspiration. Finally, thank you to those dedicating your lives to the profession of nursing. Whether you are a newly licensed nurse or a seasoned nurse or you are transitioning into practice, I hope that you find this book full of helpful information and tips.

–Connie

I want to acknowledge Cindy Thomas and Connie McIntosh for their fantastic work, creativity, and commitment to our profession. We are blessed to have their leadership.

This book is for all the nursing students and new graduates, those whom I have had the good fortune to have as my students over the past 12 years. I have enjoyed watching you all become amazing nurses and advance practice nurses. Remember to be who you are, and to be who you want to be *now*. Don't let anyone tell you what you can be or when you can be it.

I know our profession is in good hands.

–Jennifer

About the Authors

Cynthia (Cindy) M. Thomas, EdD, MS, RNc, is an associate professor at Ball State University in the School of Nursing. She teaches leadership/management courses across three nursing programs: undergraduate, RN-BSN, and graduate. Her research line focuses on the transition from student to the professional registered nurse role.

A 40-year nursing career has afforded Thomas the choice to work in many practice areas of professional nursing, including medical/surgical, orthopedics, emergency, home care, intensive care, correctional nursing, long-term care, and assisted living communities. She served 14 years in management positions and the past 16 years teaching in higher education. She has published widely on the transition from student to the professional nurse role. She volunteers her time in various organizations, including president of the Beta Rho chapter of Sigma Theta Tau International.

Thomas holds an EdD and an MS from Ball State University in Muncie, Indiana; a BSN from the University of Phoenix, San Jose, California; an ASN from Marian University, Indianapolis, Indiana; and an LPN from the Cincinnati School of Practical Nursing, Cincinnati, Ohio.

She attributes her success to the many willing and excellent mentors she has had during her career.

Constance (Connie) E. McIntosh, EdD, MBA, RN, is an assistant professor at Ball State University, School of Nursing. She serves in the undergraduate and graduate programs, teaching leadership/management and financial management. Before teaching, she was in senior leadership roles in hospitals and healthcare organizations.

McIntosh earned both undergraduate and doctorate degrees from Ball State University. Her undergraduate degree is in nursing, and her doctorate degree is in special education. She earned her master's degree in business administration from William Woods University in Fulton, Missouri.

Along with her leadership and management experience, her expertise resides in working with exceptional children, including those diagnosed with autism spectrum disorder. She has published several articles, including articles on how school nurses can better work with children with special needs.

In addition, McIntosh volunteers her time in various organizations, including the Beta Rho chapter of Sigma Theta Tau International. She has also served on the Indiana State Board of Nursing for 8 years, 3 years as president.

Jennifer S. Mensik, PhD, MBA, RN, NEA-BC, FAAN, earned a PhD in nursing from the University of Arizona College of Nursing with a major in health systems and a minor in public administration from the Eller Business College. Mensik wears many hats: She is the executive director of On Nursing Excellence and the Institute for Staffing Excellence and Innovation, as well as faculty for Arizona State University College of Nursing and Health Innovation DNP and undergraduate programs. She assists as a director of professional practice at Banner Ironwood Medical Center and Banner Goldfield Medical Center in Arizona. Mensik has authored numerous publications, including the books *Lead, Drive, & Thrive in the System* and *The Nurse Manager's Guide to Innovative Staffing.*

Mensik was employed at the three-time Magnet-designated St. Luke's Health System in Boise, Idaho, as the administrator of nursing and patient care. Before joining St. Luke's, she was the executive director of quality and patient safety for the UCLA health system. In addition, she worked at Banner Health, based in Phoenix, Arizona, in various roles, including the system director of clinical practice and research. There, she led the development of the professional nursing practice framework, which is now used in all Banner Health hospitals and has been adopted by other non-Banner Health hospitals and medical centers nationally. Mensik was named Alumni of the Year for the University of Arizona College of Nursing in 2010 and was inducted as a Fellow into the American Academy of Nursing in 2014.

Mensik has served as the president of the Arizona Nurses Association and nationally for the American Nurses Association, as second vice president on the board of directors. Additionally, she held the role of governor of nursing practice for the Western Institute of Nursing. She has published and presented nationally and regionally on quality, staffing, and professional practice.

Table of Contents

9 Looking to Practice Outside of the Hospital 139

10 Continuing Education and Advanced Degrees 157

Introduction

Having worked over 40 years as a nurse, I like to think I have seen just about everything. However, as a nurse, you will learn and see something new every single day. That is a wonderful aspect of the nursing profession.

When I started my nursing career in 1972, I graduated from an LPN program and was quite proud of my accomplishment. I worked for the next 10 years in a variety of different areas, finally landing in the ICU of a local hospital. For a long time, LPNs were given quite a bit of latitude to complete tasks, but eventually things got much tighter and LPNs were restricted from doing those same tasks. Frustration began to creep into my career, and I realized I needed to become a registered nurse (RN).

A new LPN-to-RN bridge program looked promising, so I applied and took the required math exam. I failed the exam two times. Needless to say, I was frustrated and embarrassed. I prayed about it and decided to try one more time—and passed! I was fortunate to work with outstanding RNs and nurse educators who assumed the mentor, coach, and cheerleader roles. I needed that encouragement.

It is so important to have effective mentors and coaches, but equally important to be one. You may never know the influence you may have on another person by simply exhibiting your caring nature, attitude, and willingness to help and encourage someone.

I was always encouraged by other nurses as I continued my educational path, eventually earning BSN, MS, and EdD degrees. That encouragement is what motivated me to know that I could do it. It will likely motivate you also, and you will motivate others as you gain more experience and confidence as a registered nurse.

We three authors of this book all had different educational and career paths, but we all believe we had mentors that helped us all along the way. Nurses never work alone; work to have a respectful and trusting relationship with your nurse peers. There will be many times when you need each other's support and encouragement just to get through a difficult shift, month, or year.

We want to welcome you to this book about transitioning to the professional nurse role, regardless of your current educational level, and reaching your greatest potential for yourself and your patients.

This book has several goals:

- To help you make the transition to the professional registered nurse role

- To provide a resource for information about the NCLEX, professional practice, legal and ethical issues, your state board of nursing, continuing education, and advanced practice

- To provide you with strategies to cope with and reduce stress and to avoid and eliminate violence in healthcare

- To provide an overview of the many different nursing organizations that offer continuing education credits, peer reviewed articles, and conferences for learning and networking

An Introduction to the Chapters

In Chapter 1, you will learn about the many avenues by which you can enter the nursing profession, such as the way nurses enter into practice at the level of registered nurse (RN). You can become an

RN by way of a diploma program, an associate degree, a bachelor's entry, or a master's entry into RN practice. We will discuss these various avenues of entry into practice and discuss RN residencies and options for extended employer-sponsored orientations.

In Chapter 2, we will describe the preparation effort for the National Council Licensure Exam (NCLEX), the roles and function of the state boards of nursing (BON), the State Practice Act, and your licensure and scope of nursing practice. You may be experiencing some anxiety about taking this large exam, or you may wonder whether you are adequately prepared for the exam and prepared to practice as a registered professional nurse. This chapter will give you the information you need to succeed.

Chapter 3 will help define the difference between technical and professional practice, and why that is important to know. The technical perspective is easy to define: passing medications, starting an IV, carrying out provider orders, and handling other physical and emotional aspects of caring for a patient. But you may not have thought about the professional aspects of the profession, nor what a true profession entails. Though the first two chapters discuss the definition and your legal scope of practice, this chapter will continue to build on your understanding of the RN role—specifically, the professional role.

In Chapter 4, we discuss the legal and ethical issues that nurses may encounter when working. Many legal and ethical terms and definitions will be helpful to you as a professional nurse, some of which you may already know and some that may be new to you. Nurses are confronted with ethical issues every day of their lives, but dealing with ethical issues as a professional may be different and may even challenge your personal beliefs and moral structure. This chapter will show you the laws and legal practice information that nurses must follow to maintain licensure and provide safe, quality care to patients.

Chapter 5 will discuss your role as a team member, your role as the care coordinator, different members of the team, and key tips for high-functioning teams. As an RN taking care of a patient, you will always work on a team of some sort. Healthcare teams are vital in achieving excellent patient care. Each person contributes in some way to patient care because no lone person can do it all, and no one should try. You should understand some basics about teamwork, the larger healthcare team, and your role on the team.

Chapter 6 is all about leadership. Though every RN is a leader, it may not come natural to everyone. As a new registered nurse on the unit or in the organization, you may feel that you have no place in delegating to individuals with more years of experience. It is vital to your success that you own your role as a leader and learn to delegate effectively. To help you succeed, this chapter describes the ins and outs of delegation and provides tips for you to build your leadership skills.

Chapter 7 describes various types of stress you will encounter and specifies how you can manage each one. You may have thought that graduating from college would eliminate your stress level. The reality is that stress will always be part of your life. You must learn to balance your stress.

Chapter 8 will give you the tools you need to identify and resolve violence in the workplace. Many subtypes of violence exist, and regardless of type, violence is never acceptable and never should be tolerated. Workplace violence is not new, and nursing is no exception to violence. Workplace violence in healthcare does in fact occur more often than in any other workplace environment.

Chapter 9 will provide a guide to the world outside the acute care setting. As a new RN, most of your clinical experience and exposure to nursing has been in the acute care setting. Not surprisingly, most nurses will move directly into a hospital for their first position. However, as healthcare is reformed, more positions for RNs will soon be in the settings outside acute care. In this chapter, we will touch on various options for practicing as an RN, even as a new registered nurse, outside the hospital setting.

Chapter 10 provides information about continuing your education, whether formally in an academic setting or via continuing education credits. You may not want to think about school again for a while, but healthcare is in a continual state of change that makes it necessary for nurses to remain knowledgeable of the current best practice by way of lifelong learning. This chapter will discuss the many options for nurses to continue education, including degreed and non-degreed programs and self-study via continuing education programs.

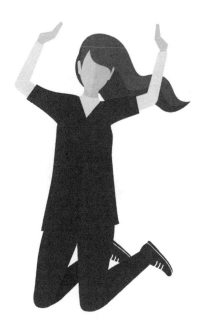

1

THE NURSING ENTRY DEGREE

ELEMENTS OF THE NURSING ENTRY DEGREE

1. Defines nursing

2. Explains the various RN entry degrees

3. Looks at the Institute of Medicine (IOM) report *The Future of Nursing: Leading Change, Advancing Health*

4. Examines Magnet-designated organizations and residency programs

5. Offers key factors when considering educational paths

Nursing is a profession of diversity. One type of diversity is the way nurses enter into practice at the registered nurse level. You can become a registered nurse (RN) in a number of ways, by completing:

- A diploma program
- An associate degree
- A bachelor's degree
- A master's entry to nursing practice (MENP)

In addition to acquiring this basic education, after you graduate and pass the National Council Licensure Examination (NCLEX), you will enter the workforce always with an orientation, but also sometimes by way of a residency program. In this chapter, we will discuss these various avenues for entry into practice, and we will describe RN residencies and the options for extended employer-sponsored orientations.

What Is Nursing?

This question may seem strange to ask of you. However, you must remember as you transition into practice what nursing is and what it should be. Our hope for you is that you will find a lifelong career in which you are capable of providing the best care possible to others. As we will discuss in later chapters (such as Chapters 4, 7, and 8), ethical, legal, and moral issues may arise that challenge you as an RN and as an individual. In those difficult times, remember why you became a nurse, and focus on what nursing should be. This strategy will guide you throughout your career as a nurse.

The American Nurses Association Definition of Nursing

Nursing is a complex profession with multiple degrees of educational preparation and an even wider variety of professional practice areas. Every nurse needs to know and understand the American Nurses Association (ANA) definition of nursing:

> Nursing *is the protection, promotion, and optimization of health and abilities, prevention of illness and injury, alleviation of suffering through the diagnosis and treatment of human response, and advocacy in the care of individuals, families, communities, and populations (ANA, 2015b).*

This definition of nursing can be applied to nurses from all levels of practice working within their scope of practice and license. Additionally, nurses have a moral and ethical responsibility to serve patients within their care regardless of race, sexual orientation, age, religion, or illness.

The ANA published a statement on the nonnegotiable code for nurses, which applies to all nurses regardless of licensure type.

The ANA *Code of Ethics for Nurses with Interpretive Statements* (or simply *Code of Ethics for Nurses*) explicates the goals, values, and ethical precepts that direct the profession of nursing (see the accompanying sidebar). The ANA believes the *Code of Ethics for Nurses* is nonnegotiable and that each nurse has an obligation to uphold and adhere to the code (ANA, 2015a).

PROVISIONS OF THE CODE OF ETHICS FOR NURSES WITH INTERPRETIVE STATEMENTS

Provision 1: The nurse practices with compassion and respect for the inherent dignity, worth, and unique attributes of every person.

Provision 2: The nurse's primary commitment is to the patient, whether an individual, family, group, community, or population.

Provision 3: The nurse promotes, advocates for, and protects the rights, health, and safety of the patient.

Provision 4: The nurse has authority, accountability, and responsibility for nursing practice; makes decisions; and takes action consistent with the obligation to promote health and to provide optimal care.

Provision 5: The nurse owes the same duties to self as to others, including the responsibility to promote health and safety, preserve wholeness of character and integrity, maintain competence, and continue personal and professional growth.

Provision 6: The nurse, through individual and collective effort, establishes, maintains, and improves the ethical environment of the work setting and conditions of employment that are conducive to safe, quality healthcare.

Provision 7: The nurse, in all roles and settings, advances the profession through research and scholarly inquiry, professional standards development, and the generation of both nursing and health policy.

Provision 8: The nurse collaborates with other health professionals and the public to protect human rights, promote health diplomacy, and reduce health disparities.

Provision 9: The profession of nursing, collectively through its professional organizations, must articulate nursing values, maintain the integrity of the profession, and integrate principles of social justice into nursing and health policy.

(ANA, 2015a)

Reviewing the Educational Entries to RN Work

As you transition into the workforce, you will work with many wonderful nurses from a variety of educational backgrounds—diploma, associate, bachelor's, and master's entry prepared RNs. Though differences exist in course work among these degrees, all programs have a similar core of courses required by national accrediting bodies such as the National League for Nursing (NLN) and the American Association of Colleges of Nursing (AACN). These core courses prepare all students to sit for and take the national certifying exam, the NCLEX. Each state board of nursing, however, oversees this process, as well as the required minimum passing score to become licensed as an RN. The NCLEX is a way to ensure that all RNs have a similar minimum knowledge base and are deemed safe to practice.

Though all RNs start somewhere, that start shouldn't always be considered the end. Your entry into practice degree may be nearing the end, or may even be finished, but that shouldn't mean you won't ever go back to school, either. In Chapter 10, we will discuss those options. The following sections will review the history of, and discuss relevant information on, several RN entry degrees. As you make these decisions, it is helpful to understand the history of nursing education and where we are headed in the future!

The Diploma Degree

The diploma degree that took two or three years to complete was once a prominent entry for many RNs.

These are the characteristics of the diploma degree path:

- This was an apprenticeship-like program, attached primarily to hospitals as a way to train their own staffs.

- As nursing evolved and transitioned into a profession, more nursing programs at the community college and university level were opening or expanding, and these programs were viewed as a more favorable type of nursing education.

- The typical diploma program gave few to no transferrable college credits.

- This program type accounts for less than 10% of nursing entry programs in the United States (AACN, 2011).

 DID YOU KNOW?

In the 1980s, approximately 55% of RNs held the diploma degree as their highest level of nursing education. By 2008, that percentage had dropped to 13.9% of all RNs (AACN, 2011).

The Associate Degree

The associate degree in nursing (ADN/ASN) is an effective way to enter into the professional nursing practice and transition to the baccalaureate degree.

The 2-year associate degree program was conceived in the 1940s because of a registered nurse decline during the World War II period. The first program was developed in 1952 by Fairleigh Dickinson University in New Jersey. Most ADN/ASN programs were in community colleges, where enrollment continued to increase until the 1990s, when the ADN/ASN was considered to be more of a transition to the bachelor of science in nursing (BSN) (Bender, 2015).

The Fairleigh Dickinson University School of Nursing associate degree program graduated its last class in 1970 and was replaced by the generic baccalaureate program (Fairleigh Dickinson University, 2015).

These are the characteristics of the associate degree path:

- Generally, the ADN/ASN degree may be completed within 2 years in addition to prerequisite coursework (3 years).

- Associate degreed nurses take the same National Council Licensure Examination (NCLEX) as the BSN-prepared nurse, reflecting minimal competency that all registered nurses must be able to demonstrate.

- Employment for associate degreed nurses continues to be good because there continues to be a nursing shortage; however, practice environments may be more limited than those for BSN-prepared nurses.

- There is a nationwide movement pushing toward 80% of all RNs to be BSN-prepared by 2020. Many employers, especially Magnet hospitals and those on the Magnet-designation journey, may hire only BSN-prepared RNs.

We will talk more about Magnet-designated healthcare organizations later in this chapter. Knowing this information may help you with future career planning.

 DID YOU KNOW?

The United States has 692 RN-to-BSN and 159 RN-to-MSN accredited programs (AACN, 2014b).

REFLECTION

I started my nursing career as a licensed practical nurse (LPN). I had a great nursing foundation on which to build. After working for 10 years I began to get weary of the limitations placed on me and decided to apply to an LPN bridge associate degree program (ASN) at a local college. A specific score on a math exam was a mandatory part of the entrance requirements. Two times I missed the required score by one point. I was really frustrated and almost gave up but decided to try one more time. Finally, on the third try I passed the math exam. Never give up if it is something you really want to do. A nursing degree is worth the fight.

–Cindy Thomas, EdD, MS, RNc

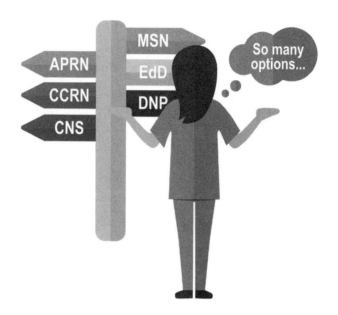

The Bachelor's Degree

We want you to have a good understanding of why more and more organizations are requiring nurses to have the BSN to be hired. Nurse researchers such as Amos (2015) explain that the constant changes in healthcare are creating the need for better educated and prepared registered nurses who can function in outpatient-type environments such as surgical centers, home care locations, clinics, schools, and community centers.

This change in practice environments forces the nursing profession to reevaluate the bachelor's degree (BSN) as the entry-level degree for registered nurses. The BSN should be not only the entry degree but also the initial degree from which nurses eventually build a career by pursuing graduate-level study for advanced practice roles (Amos, 2015).

These are the characteristics of the bachelor's degree path:

- The traditional BSN is a 4-year accredited college/ university degree that incorporates liberal arts courses in addition to professional education and training for high school graduates or individuals with no previous nursing education (Amos, 2015).

- The United States now has approximately 700 BSN accredited programs.

- Baccalaureate degreed nurses are educated to develop good communication skills, critical thinking and reasoning, and leadership and management attributes.

- Differing from associate degree (ASN) programs, BSN degree curriculums require courses such as community health, leadership and management, and research. Students are placed in a wider variety of clinical settings such as schools, public and community programs, clinics, and social service agencies, preparing BSN nurses to practice in all environments (AACN, 2000; Amos, 2015).

- The AACN (2015) declares that entry-level-prepared nurses must have an increased knowledge of community-based primary healthcare and place an importance on health promotion, health maintenance, and cost-effective quality care.

A great deal of research takes place around BSN-prepared RNs, and you should know your facts on this degree (see the accompanying sidebar).

INTERESTING FACTS ABOUT BSN NURSES

Patient outcomes improve with more BSN nurses (Kutney-Lee, Sloane, and Aiken, 2013).

BSN-prepared nurses have a higher nurse job satisfaction (ANA, 2013).

Post-surgery patient mortality rates decrease when more BSN-prepared nurses are present (Kutney-Lee, Sloane, and Aiken, 2013).

Military nursing requires a BSN as the entry level (ANA, 2013).

More employers are seeking BSN nurses (AACN, 2010).

A BSN is a move closer to a master's degree (*Scrubs,* 2015).

BSN-prepared nurses generally earn higher salaries (*Scrubs,* 2015).

Greater employment opportunities are available for BSN-prepared nurses (*Scrubs,* 2015).

BSN nurses make up 55% of all nurses since 2013 (AACN, 2014a).

The University of Minnesota was the first BSN program in the United States (Bender, 2015).

REFLECTION

After I earned an associate degree (ASN) and worked for another 10 years, I got the urge to earn a baccalaureate degree (BSN). This is significant because I always said I would never earn a BSN, and if I did go back to school, I would earn a degree in a different field. (My advice: Never say that.) I applied and got accepted and, after earning a BSN degree, immediately entered a master's degree program. I was on a path of no return as I eventually earned a doctorate. I have learned that education opens doors for more opportunities. You can never have too much education.

–Cindy Thomas, EdD, MS, RNc

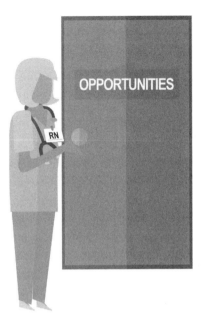

The Master's Entry to Nursing Practice (MENP)

The master's entry to nursing practice is a unique entry degree.

These are the characteristics of the master's entry to nursing practice degree path:

- Though you can find BSN acceleration programs, for individuals who already hold a bachelor's degree in another field and want to move into nursing, this is similar.

- Some confusion surrounds this role and its degree, assuming that a master's degree in nursing is an automatic advance practice role. Some of the master's entry programs are designed to result in an advanced practice RN degree such as a nurse practitioner (NP) role, whereas others result in an entry RN role.

- Those who choose to enter into this as an entry RN program all have bachelor's degrees from other fields and would rather not obtain another bachelor's degree.

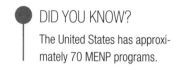

DID YOU KNOW?
The United States has approximately 70 MENP programs.

Many online and ground programs (in physical buildings) offer exciting opportunities for RNs seeking to return to college to earn advanced degrees.

An *online* nursing program is offered through your computer. You use the Internet to access the program and its course content and then to submit your completed assignments. Online programs can be valuable methods for many nurses who seek advanced education but who live in more remote areas or lack access to a ground campus. Online programs also offer great flexibility, allowing you to access the courses anywhere in the world as long as you have Internet access and at any time, day or night. This method of learning is attractive to many working students.

Many ground colleges and universities now offer advanced degree programs online. If you are self-motivated and do not need physical, face-to-face contact, you may be well-suited for an online program.

Some benefits of online programs are that courses can be accessed from anywhere in the world and at any time, they don't interfere with work schedules, and they're completed in a safe home environment. Some drawbacks of online programs are that their tuition cost is often higher, you will experience a lack of personal connection to others, you will need to be self-directed, and programs may or may not offer a traditional graduation ceremony.

A *ground* nursing program is in a physical building or on a college/ university campus. Ground nursing programs are located in almost every state in the United States and other countries around the world. A ground educational experience is also a valuable way to earn an advanced degree, as the program faculty meet face to face in actual classrooms. If you prefer the standard method of physical interaction with faculty and other students, a ground educational experience might be a great option.

The benefits of a ground campus program are physical interaction with others, a traditional college/university environment, established days and times for classes, and a traditional graduation ceremony. Potential drawbacks are drive time to classes, conflicts between class schedules and work schedules, the cost of fuel for driving, and safety considerations if commuting at night.

Examining the Institute of Medicine's The Future of Nursing Report

One of the most respected and embraced documents on nursing education of our times, the Institute of Medicine's (IOM) report *The Future of Nursing: Leading Change, Advancing Health*, was published in 2010. This report has four key messages that led to further recommendations:

1. Nurses should practice to the full extent of their education and training.

2. Nurses should achieve higher levels of education and training by way of an improved education system that promotes seamless academic progression.

3. Nurses should be full partners with physicians and other health professionals in redesigning healthcare in the United States.

4. Effective workforce planning and policy making require better data collection and an improved information infrastructure (IOM, 2011).

The second recommendation, to achieve higher levels of education, has prompted the recommendation that 80% of RNs be BSN-prepared by 2020. The Robert Wood Johnson Foundation and many other nursing organizations have partnered in every state to create action coalitions to achieve this goal.

Accomplishing this goal requires a multipronged approach. This doesn't mean that diploma and ADN/ASN programs will no longer exist. Many states have started or improved on the bridge between these degrees and the BSN.

THE FUTURE OF NURSING

We highly suggest that you visit the website http://www.thefutureofnursing.org to learn more about action coalition work in your state.

Considering Your Employment Opportunities

As you transition from education into practice, you may experience panic, worry, and confusion setting in regarding employment opportunities. Accepting a new position is always stressful. To be successful, go online and read about the local job market for RNs in your city or in the city where you want to get a position. Some areas and states in the United States have RN shortages, and some have an oversupply.

DID YOU KNOW?

The average first-year turnover for new RNs is 30%—or, stated another way, 30% of new RNs will leave their unit or place of employment within one year (AACN, 2014c).

Though you need to consider many issues, we will discuss here the ones with a bigger impact on you professionally.

Employment Settings

According to the United States Bureau of Labor Statistics, approximately 61% of RNs worked in a hospital setting in 2012 (2015). We will talk more about employment and various settings in Chapter 10, but as you read this book, think outside the box about this topic. With changes in the healthcare environment, the Affordable Care Act, and Accountable Care Organizations, a real shift is taking place from inpatient to outpatient settings that is already prompting these settings to hire and recruit new registered nurses.

Magnet-Designated Organizations

You may have had the luck to have had a clinical rotation in an American Nurses Credentialing Center (ANCC) Magnet-designated hospital or healthcare organization. This is a specific designation from the ANCC, a subsidiary of the American Nurses Association (ANA) that recognizes hospitals and healthcare organizations that provide nursing excellence. This is the highest and most prestigious international distinction.

As of March 2015, 410 hospitals worldwide have received this designation (ANCC, 2015). Any healthcare organization that employs RNs may apply for and achieve this distinction — it is not for hospitals only. This nursing distinction is one to consider when you are evaluating various employers.

Registered Nurse Residency Programs

Lastly in this chapter, we want to discuss residency programs. The word *residency* gets thrown around a lot, so it is important to understand what this concept is in relation to entry RN practice. There is no one-model-fits-all in regard to a definition of residency because different employers (normally, hospitals) have created their own programs for RNs transitioning into practice for the first time. Residency programs are designed to partner continued education with work experience to support new RNs in their first year of practice. A residency program can be anywhere from 3 to 12 months long.

 DID YOU KNOW?

Research outcomes on a single yearlong residency program found retention rates of 94.3% for RNs in their first year (AACN, 2014c).

The *Future of Nursing* report also noted nursing residencies as one of its key recommendations:

> *Recommendation 3: Implement nurse residency programs. State boards of nursing, accrediting bodies, the federal government, and healthcare organizations should take actions to support nurses' completion of a transition-to-practice program (nurse residency) after they have completed a prelicensure or advanced practice degree program or when they are transitioning into new clinical practice areas (IOM, 2011).*

The IOM report notes that state boards of nursing and accrediting bodies should support nurse residencies for both RN and advanced practice registered nurses (APRNs). Additionally, the IOM report states that healthcare organizations that currently provide nurse residencies should evaluate the effectiveness in improving the retention of nurses, expanding competencies, and improving patient outcomes (IOM, 2011).

Though it is advantageous to attend a nurse residency program, not many organizations have one. Follow these strategies to find a nurse residency program:

- While you are interviewing, talk to the hiring manager about orientation, and see whether it includes a residency.

- Talk to your nursing advisor.

- Check with past nursing graduates. (They can be helpful resources!)

- Search organization websites to learn more about the potential for a residency program before your interview.

EXPERIENCE FROM THE FIELD: MY PERSONAL JOURNEY FROM ADN TO BSN

I was born into a family that had never attended college. My family had its share of police officers, craftsmen, and business owners, so hard work, not education, was my heritage. I worked in my family's business early on and learned the carpentry trade, but it was not right for me. I longed for education and science and to make our society better.

Although it was difficult to leave my family's business, I knew that nursing was the right profession for me. I enrolled at Lane Community College's Associate of Applied Science in Nursing program. I quickly became involved in nonprofit leadership and volunteer coordination. My community college nursing program was incredibly diverse, with people from all walks of life. I greatly appreciated being able to collaborate with students who had been journalists, engineers, linguists, and nursing assistants. My associate's degree equipped me with the skills to excel at bedside nursing, and I found a staff nurse position quickly, though it still felt as though my education was incomplete.

I immediately enrolled in Oregon Health and Science University's RN to BSN program. From my work with the National Student Nurses Association and the American Nurses Association, I felt that I needed the critical thinking and leadership skills that a BSN offered in order to truly make an impact on the health of my community. Practicing as a licensed RN while I studied for a BSN also allowed me to provide monetarily for my family.

I chose to utilize my bedside nursing skills as an asset to my pursuit of a BSN. I was able to use RN skills on a daily basis as I learned leadership skills to augment my practice. The RN-to-BSN community brought many different types of people with unique perspectives that helped me to more fully develop my own understanding of problems and to think outside of the box for solutions.

Though the path from RN to BSN was longer, I chose it so that I could maintain balance in my family life. As a husband and father of two young children, I wanted to be certain that I could still be a dad while pursuing my education and practicing as an RN. The best thing about nursing is that there are so many specialties and a great need for nurses from every background to help solve the healthcare problems of the future and to provide the best care possible for our diverse patient population.

–Jesse Kennedy, RN

Deciding What Educational Path Works for You

Each person has a personal journey and a professional journey. At various points in your life, you will need to make decisions that will affect both. If you want to go back to school, particularly for your BSN, consider these factors:

1. **Hospitals and healthcare organizations prefer RNs with BSNs as opposed to a different type of bachelor's degree.** Though you may want to diversify your education, consider the BSN the minimum professional degree.

2. **Organizations that are on the Magnet journey or Magnet designated are working toward higher numbers of BSN-prepared staff.** A bachelor's degree in another field does not count.

3. **There are many different online and ground programs.** Think about how you do your best learning. After you start a program, it may not be easy to transfer credits.

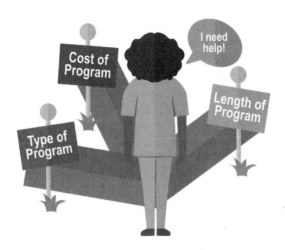

4. **If you view an exclusively online model as acceptable for your continuing education, you open up the possibilities on the number of schools you can attend.** You do not need to attend only a local or in-state school.

5. **Consider length of time.** RN-to-BSN programs differ in length depending on whether the program offers a schedule of one class or multiple classes at a time.

6. **Consider price.** Though one university may have an easier, shorter program, it may also be more expensive.

7. **Consider the reputation of the university and the college/school of nursing.** Not all universities are equal. The place where you get your degree serves as your pedigree. No, we aren't saying that you need to go to an Ivy League school, but various ranking/rating systems are out there for colleges. Take the time to get to know the school you may attend before you apply to the program.

As you begin your career as an RN, you should know the different educational entry points of fellow colleagues. You should also recognize the importance of continuing your education if you have not yet obtained a bachelor's degree in nursing. As you continue in your transition, remember the definition of nursing, and remember the foundation of your nursing education. This definition, with the ANA *Code of Ethics for Nurses*, will be your guide in any situation you may encounter.

Chapter Checkup

These are the key points from this chapter:

❑ Nursing is a profession of diversity.

❑ Every nurse should know and understand the American Nurses Association (ANA) definition of nursing.

❑ The ANA published a statement on the nonnegotiable *Code of Ethics for Nurses*, which applies to all nurses regardless of licensure type.

❑ The IOM report *The Future of Nursing* notes that "nurses should achieve higher levels of education and training through an improved education system that promotes seamless academic progression" and has set a key goal of 80% of all RNs as BSN level or higher by 2020.

❑ Look at Magnet-designated healthcare organizations as preferred settings for employment. These organizations are more likely to also have extensive residency programs.

❑ Consider the many aspects of online and traditional ground nursing programs before you decide what program works best for your lifestyle and your work and family needs.

References

American Association of Colleges of Nursing (AACN). (2000). The baccalaureate degree in nursing as minimal preparation for professional practice. Retrieved from http://www.aacn.nche.edu/publications/position/bacc-degree-prep

American Association of Colleges of Nursing (AACN). (2010). Your nursing career: A look at the facts. Retrieved from http://www.aacn.nche.edu/students/your-nursing-career/facts

American Association of Colleges of Nursing (AACN). (2011). Nursing fact sheet. Retrieved from http://www.aacn.nche.edu/media-relations/fact-sheets/nursing-fact-sheet

American Association of Colleges of Nursing (AACN). (2014a). Creating a more highly qualified nursing workforce. Retrieved from http://www.aacn.nche.edu/media-relations/fact-sheets/nursing-workforce

American Association of Colleges of Nursing (AACN). (2014b). The impact of education on nursing practice. Retrieved from http://www.aacn.nche.edu/media-relations/fact-sheets/impact-of-education_

American Association of Colleges of Nursing (AACN). (2014c). Nurse residency programs. Retrieved from http://www.aacn.nche.edu/education-resources/nurse-residency-program

American Association of Colleges of Nursing (AACN). (2015). The baccalaureate degree in nursing as minimal preparation for professional practice. Retrieved from http://www.aacn.nche.edu/publications/position/bacc-degree-prep

American Nurses Association (ANA). (2013). Nursing education. Retrieved from http://www.nursingworld.org/MainMenuCategories/Policy-Advocacy/State/Legislative-Agenda-Reports/NursingEducation

American Nurses Association (ANA). (2015a). Code of ethics for nurses with interpretive statements. Retrieved from http://www.nursingworld.org/MainMenuCategories/EthicsStandards/CodeofEthicsforNurses/Code-of-Ethics-For-Nurses.html

American Nurses Association (ANA). (2015b). What is nursing? Retrieved from http://www.nursingworld.org/EspeciallyForYou/What-is-Nursing

American Nurses Credentialing Center (ANCC). (2015). Frequently asked questions about ANCC's Magnet Recognition Program. Retrieved from http://www.nurse-credentialing.org/Magnet/International/MagnetProgOverview/MagnetProgFAQ.aspx

Amos, L. K. (2015). Baccalaureate nursing programs. Retrieved from http://www.aacn.nche.edu/education-resources/bsn-article

Bender, J. (2015). Associate's degrees in nursing: The road ahead. Retrieved from http://www.bestnursingdegree.com/adn-to-bsn

Bureau of Labor Statistics, U.S. Department of Labor. (2014). *Occupational Outlook Handbook*, 2014-15 Edition, Registered Nurses. Retrieved from http://www.bls.gov/ooh/healthcare/registered-nurses.htm

Fairleigh Dickinson University. (2015). The Henry P. Becton School of Nursing and Allied Health. Retrieved from http://view2.fdu.edu/academics/university-college/school-of-nursing-and-allied-health

Institute of Medicine (IOM). (2011). *The future of nursing: Leading change, advancing health*. Washington, DC: The National Academies Press.

Kutney-Lee, A., Sloane, D. M., & Aiken, L. H. (2013). An increase in the number of nurses with baccalaureate degrees is linked to lower rates of post-surgery mortality. *Health Affairs, 32*(3), 579–586.

Scrubs. (2015). 12 biggest reasons nurses get a BSN. Retrieved from http://scrubsmag.com/12-biggest-reasons-nurses-get-a-bsn

PREPARING FOR THE NCLEX AND YOUR LICENSE

ELEMENTS OF PREPARING FOR THE NCLEX AND YOUR LICENSE

1. Examines the NCLEX

2. Discusses preparing for the exam

3. Prepares you to register for the NCLEX

4. Weighs the pros and cons of retaking the exam

5. Discusses state boards of nursing

In this chapter we discuss your preparation for the National Council Licensure Exam (NCLEX), the roles and function of the state boards of nursing, the state practice act, and your licensure and scope of nursing practice. You may be experiencing some anxiety about taking a lengthy exam, and you may even wonder whether you are adequately prepared for the exam and prepared to practice as a registered professional nurse.

Stop. Take a deep breath, and consider all your preparation efforts over the past several years while in a nursing program. You know far more than you think you do about preparing for this exam, and we want to give you some helpful information about the NCLEX.

We will discuss the many resources available to help you review for the NCLEX. We recommend that you do everything possible to be well prepared before scheduling your time to take the NCLEX.

Also, until now you may have had no idea what a state board of nursing does or how the board is directly related to the NCLEX or how the state board supports nurses. This chapter will also explain state nurse practice acts and help to define the license and scope of practice for the registered nurse (RN).

You are about to take (arguably) the most important exam of your life. Passing this exam allows for your licensure application, so you should understand all areas of the exam.

Preparing for the NCLEX

The NCLEX is the licensing exam for nurses in the United States and Canada (NCSBNa, 2014). There are two types of exams:

- NCLEX-RN, to become a registered nurse, or RN

- NCLEX-PN, to become a licensed practical nurse, or LPN
  (NCSBNa, 2014)

Students who earn a nursing degree from, and successfully graduate from, an associate degree program (2-year), a diploma program (3-year), or a baccalaureate program (4-year) will take the
NCLEX-RN. To ensure public safety, each state board of nursing
requires that anyone wanting to practice nursing must successfully
pass the NCLEX-RN, which tests minimum competency for an
entry-level nurse (NCSBN, 2014a). You must pass this licensure
exam before applying for licensure in the state in which you want
to practice.

Who Owns the NCLEX?

The National Council of State Boards of Nursing (NCSBN) is a
professional organization that consists of all 50 states' boards of
nursing. It is the NCSBN that developed and owns the NCLEX
(NCSBN, 2014a).

Before you take the NCLEX-RN test, visit the many resources located on the
NCSBN website, including the frequently asked questions (FAQ) sheet (NCSBN,
2014b). Resources include an application for the exam, registration, and the overall test plan. Reading, reviewing, and familiarizing yourself with these resources is
a vital part of the preparation.

Whether you are a new graduate or you have recently moved to a
state that requires licensure applicants to take the NCLEX-RN,
preparation for the examination is *essential*—we cannot stress it
enough. Every nurse must successfully pass the NCLEX in order
to be licensed. This exam can provoke anxiety. Understanding the

examination process can help you lower the anxiety you feel on exam day.

The NCLEX-RN is a *computer adaptive test (CAT)*, in which each candidate exam is created as each question is answered. If the candidate answers the question correctly, the test bank is queried for a more difficult question to answer. If the candidate incorrectly answers the question, an easier question is offered.

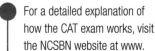 For a detailed explanation of how the CAT exam works, visit the NCSBN website at www. ncsbn.org.

These are the key characteristics of the NCLEX-RN:

- Because of the individuality of the CAT, no two candidates will receive the same NCLEX-RN.

- You must answer the question that is presented; skipping questions is not permitted.

- There is no penalty for guessing on questions that you might find unfamiliar.

- All candidates will have to answer at least 75 questions, which is the minimum number of questions.

- Of the 75 questions, 60 questions will be from the NCLEX-RN test bank. The other 15 are *pretest* questions: The NCSBN is testing them for future exams. These pretest questions do not count in your overall NCLEX score.

What Content Is on the NCLEX?

Content knowledge was introduced, covered, and reinforced during your educational experience. Schools of nursing curriculum are designed to properly cover the various patient needs and how to prepare for medication administration, interventions, and medical treatment. For example, you likely were required to take a course in foundational nursing, which included both didactic and clinical requirements. Foundational nursing will likely be covered on the NCLEX-RN as a client need of *Physiological Integrity: Basic Care and Comfort.*

The NCLEX-RN test plan outlines the four client needs that are covered on the examination itself (NCSBN, 2012):

- Health promotion and maintenance
- Psychosocial integrity
- Safe and effective care environment
- Physiological integrity (NCLEX-RN Test Plan, 2012)

Two of the four categories (safe and effective care environment and physiological integrity) contain subcategories including management of care, safety and infection control, basic care and comfort, pharmacological and parenteral therapies, reduction of risk therapies, and physiological adaptation (NCLEX-RN Test Plan, 2012).

The NCLEX-RN Test Plan (2012) provides important information regarding content distribution within the examination itself. For example, the NCLEX-RN Test Plan indicates the questions related to safe and effective care environment (management of care) will be between 17% and 23% of the overall test.

Using a Review Manual

In addition to identifying the client areas covered by the exam itself, test takers can read an NCLEX-RN review manual. These manuals, published by various companies, review major content areas for nursing, including fundamentals, maternity, pediatric, adult medical-surgical, critical care, and mental health.

These review manuals typically offer content chapter assessments (i.e., sample test questions). Reviewing sample test questions can help you identify areas of strength and weakness related to the various content areas. For example, if maternity is an area of strength for you, you may choose instead to focus on an area where you have less knowledge.

Taking a Review Course

You also may choose to prepare for the examination by attending an *organized review* course, which is offered online or onsite. If the review course is onsite, it typically lasts a few days. This type of course offers an evaluation of your strengths and weaknesses in each of the core content areas. In addition, an organized review course typically offers test-taking suggestions, including how to identify the stem of the NCLEX question. This identification allows you to focus on what the question is asking, therefore easily eliminating distractors in the available answer options. (See the sample NCLEX question in the nearby sidebar.)

Preparing Physically for the Exam

Following similar test-preparation strategies as you did for your college exams will also benefit you in preparing for the NCLEX. Establishing healthy eating and wellness habits can go a long way toward exam success, as described in these examples:

- To help decrease the chance of pre-exam illness, eat a healthy diet while varying meals.

- Incorporate regular exercise into your routine to lower your stress level as the exam draws nearer.

- Get plenty of rest, including the age-recommended amount of sleep, to eliminate tiredness during the exam itself and allow you to focus.

SAMPLE NCLEX QUESTION

The nurse discovers he made a medication error for one of his patients today. No one else witnessed the error or knows about it. To follow ethical standards, the nurse should:

(Select all that apply)

1. Do nothing.

2. Write and submit an incident report on himself.

3. Notify the patient's physician of the error.

4. Notify the patient's family of the error.

Answers: 2 and 3

Rationale:

#1: This answer is incorrect because nurses must self-report all incidents regardless of whether other people witnessed them. Self-reporting is also a part of following proper ethical standards.

#2: Nurses must work within an ethical framework. Even though no one witnessed the nurse make the error, the error still occurred. The incident report will help the risk management committee determine why and how the error was made and how to prevent it from happening again.

#3: The physician must be notified of the medication error to determine whether the medication should be given late or whether to make further changes in the medication schedule.

#4: This answer is incorrect because it is not necessary to notify the patient's family. However, the patient would need to be informed after the physician has determined whether changes will be made to the medication schedule.

Sleep is an important part of living a healthy and productive lifestyle. Sleeping is the brain's way to digest and retain the materials you have learned. Carey (2014) discussed how the first half of the night's sleep is the retention period, and the second half is the motor memory consolidation period. Therefore, missing sleep is like missing this time for your brain to process information. Harris Health System (2015) mentioned that being well rested can improve memory recall and the ability to maintain concentration. Getting a good night of sleep can help you remember information more easily.

Similarly, rapid eye movement, know as *REM sleep*, helps with deciphering hidden patterns, comprehending, and seeing solutions to difficult problems (Carey, 2014). Getting sufficient rest can be helpful for learning and retaining information you have studied. Harris Health System (2015) suggests that individuals in their early twenties should, ideally, sleep 8 or 9 hours every night. Students typically do not get sufficient hours of sleep, and it can affect their concentration, learning, and academic performance (Harris Health System, 2015). Pairing a good night of sleep with effective study habits can increase the likelihood of performing well on the exam.

Cramming for the NCLEX?

A common misconception about studying is that *cramming* (studying intensively) the night before a test is effective. In reality, losing sleep by cramming for a test is found to be less effective than spreading out study time and getting enough sleep (Prometric, 2014). Because the NCLEX tests a wide range of course content, cramming is not recommended. In fact, you have been learning the course content throughout your entire nursing curriculum. Therefore, attempting to "learn" the material days before the exam is counterproductive. Rather, you should study for a set amount of time (perhaps an hour) every day over the course of a few weeks before the exam. This strategy gives your brain the opportunity to truly learn and retain the information.

Where Should I Study and Prepare?

Consistently using the same study environment that is conducive to focusing is essential in test preparation. Dorm rooms, living rooms, or coffee shops can be suitable for some people but are often filled with distractors. TV, roommates, background noises, and even one's own children can all be distracting when trying to focus on studying.

Finding a quiet place to study and eliminating distractions is the key to creating a more effective study environment (Grohol, 2006).

Simulating the test-taking environment may assist with your preparation for the NCLEX. Therefore, removing distractors such as Facebook, Twitter, and Netflix can be helpful. To eliminate the temptation of doing something else, bring only those items that are necessary for studying.

Frequent Breaks From Studying Are Good

Because studying requires a great deal of focus, be sure to take breaks and reward yourself (Grohol, 2006). Taking breaks while studying is a good habit to create. Setting rewards such as letting yourself watch an episode of your favorite show after finishing a chapter can help motivate you to study. Breaks and rewards can also keep you from becoming overwhelmed or worn out.

Prometric (2014) suggests studying using a variety of different techniques, such as reading books, completing practice tests, and watching instructional videos. Using a variety of study techniques allows for different types of learning and can also prevent you from becoming bored while studying.

In addition to practicing typical studying habits, you should study with the right mind-set. Trying to study with a negative mind-set can make it quite difficult to determine which information is important. Grohol (2006) suggests trying to think positively about your skills and abilities while studying.

Grohol also recommends avoiding catastrophic thinking, such as, "I will never have enough time to study," and absolute thinking, such as, "I always screw things up for myself." Grohol (2006) suggests that, rather than think these kinds of thoughts, you recognize that perhaps you did not have much time or did not do as well as you wanted, but that if you focus and study, you can still do your best. Catastrophic thinking, again, is merely distracting you from truly studying. Overall, having the right mind-set, environment, and study techniques can result in effective standardized test preparation.

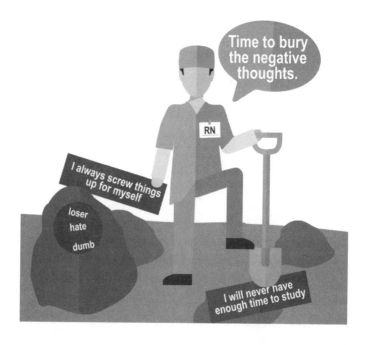

Finding the Exam Site

The last thing you want to do is miss your exam time. Therefore, eliminate all possible causes of missing the exam time:

- Before you do anything else, print the directions to the exam site. Do not count on mapping apps on your phone to get you to the exam site. If your phone battery dies, you will not have directions easily on hand.

- Days before the exam, physically make a test run to the exam site. Take note of how long it takes you to arrive at the exam site.

- Plan to go early. Gas up your vehicle the night before, therefore eliminating the need to make unnecessary stops on the day of the test.

Being Prepared on Exam Day

Along with preparation strategies leading up to the day of your standardized test are helpful tips for being prepared when exam day arrives.

First, eat a healthy breakfast. Many individuals seem to skip this meal; however, you should eat a suitable meal in the morning (Prometric, 2014). Scholastic (2015) explained that skipping breakfast to sleep can make you more tired than if you had woken up and eaten breakfast. This meal can provide you with energy to focus and recall information for the test. Fruit, oatmeal, wheat toast, yogurt, and eggs are all healthy options for a good breakfast on test day (Scholastic, 2015).

Snacks can also be important during standardized tests. Some tests allow for breaks during which you can use the restroom or grab a quick snack. Peanut butter with apple slices, cheese cubes, fruit, raw vegetables, and nuts are all examples of healthy snacks for keeping up your energy and focus during a standardized test (Scholastic, 2015).

Before taking the test, use the restroom and organize your supplies to ensure that you have everything you need before getting started (Prometric, 2014). Doing so can alleviate the stress of realizing that you are missing a needed supply halfway through the exam.

During the exam, go back and review your responses. Prometric (2014) mentioned that although people often say to "trust your gut," you should review your answers to make sure that you have made the correct choices.

Also, when you are working through the test, skip questions that you feel stressed about and return to them later. This way, you can prevent your stress level from affecting other questions to which you know the answers. As you review your test to double-check your answers, you can also respond to those that you did not answer originally. Take deep breaths and remain focused in order to reduce your stress level (Prometric, 2014).

REGISTERING FOR THE NCLEX EXAM

Registering for the exam is an important part of the NCLEX process. Detailed information on registration is on the NCSBN website at www.ncsbn.org. The costs associated with the exam are also highlighted.

What to Do if You Fail the NCLEX Exam

Candidates who do not pass the examination will be provided with results on how they performed in each of the content areas. The results come in the form of a document known as the *NCLEX*

Candidate Performance Results (CPR). Candidates are encouraged to use the CPR when studying for their next retake (NCSBN, 2014a).

Candidates who want to retake the examination will need to contact their individual boards of nursing. The individual state boards of nursing (BON) may have specific statutes, or regulations, that limit the number of times a candidate may attempt the exam.

In addition, candidates retaking the exam must wait between 45 and 90 days until taking the next exam. After gaining BON clearance, the candidate will need to reregister for the examination with the test administrator and pay the fee. In addition, the candidate will receive a new Authorized To Test (ATT). After you receive the new ATT, you can schedule your exam.

EXPERIENCE FROM THE FIELD

Those of us who work as school of nursing faculty strive to prepare students to take the NCLEX. That preparation goes beyond the obvious nursing content and clinical skills. We review test-taking skills with our students. And we drive home the importance of adequate rest, refining study skills, and establishing a study routine. I can't tell you the number of times I've had candidates (former students) report back after taking the NCLEX that they wished they had followed my instructions because I was exactly right and on target with my test preparation tips and hints. Two of the best preparation tips we encourage: Take hundreds or thousands of NCLEX practice test questions, and attend a formal NCLEX test review.

—Constance E. McIntosh, EdD, MBA, RN

Understanding State Boards of Nursing, Your License, and Scope of Practice

Nursing licensure is regulated by the state board of nursing (BON). The BON is a member of the larger National Council of

State Boards of Nursing (NCSBN, 2014a). Although driven by different state policies, BONs share a common mission of public safety and protection while advocating for the public by effectively regulating the practice of nursing.

BONs are responsible for licensure of the nurses within each state. Applicants for licensure may come from new nursing graduates needing to successfully pass the NCLEX-RN or from RNs who are transferring from one state to another. A nurse must have a valid state license in order to practice in an individual state.

The *nurse practice act* is a state's dynamic document that addresses the responsibilities of RNs and their scope of practice. The ANA describes the scope of practice as the "who, what, where, when, why, and how" of nursing practice (ANA, 2012). Every state has a nurse practice act, which is enacted by each state's legislature. Because nursing encompasses a large set of clinical and professional skills, it would be impossible for any nurse practice act to address every professional situation that may occur within the course of a career (Russell, 2012). Therefore, it is up to the individual's state BON to interpret the nurse practice act while developing rules and regulations that will help the RN when making decisions in care delivery.

The BON authority is not limited to licensure issues and nurse practice act oversight. The BON is also responsible for the education standards for schools of nursing. Schools of nursing must receive initial and ongoing accreditation from the BON. When compliance of these education standards is not met or maintained, accreditation can be pulled, leading to the closing of schools.

As an RN, you are encouraged to know your state's nurse practice act. The NCSBN has developed a helpful resource — the nurse practice act toolkit. The toolkit offers an increased understanding of each state's regulations and is a guide to how to locate each state's act.

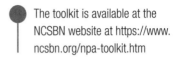 The toolkit is available at the NCSBN website at https://www. ncsbn.org/npa-toolkit.htm

Every nurse should understand what role the state board of nursing plays in relation to his or her own license. Every state has a nurse practice act, and the nurse will be required to practice within the guidelines of the individual state's act. Before applying for licensure in any state, take the time to review the application for licensure, the guidelines, the state's practice act, and any requirements, such as continuing education units, needed for unencumbered licensure.

Chapter Checkup

Key points from this chapter include:

- ❏ The NCLEX is a licensing exam for nursing program graduates in the United States and Canada.

- ❏ The NCLEX indicates the minimal competency of the new registered nurse.

- ❏ Register for the NCLEX in the state where you plan to practice nursing.

- ❏ Every state in the United States has a nurse practice act.

- ❏ Review online or visit your individual state board of nursing so that you understand what role the board plays for registered nurses.

- ❏ A registered nurse license must be renewed according to individual state board of nursing rules.

References

American Nurses Association (ANA). (2012). *Nursing: Scope and standards of practice* (2nd edition). Silver Spring, MD: Author.

Carey, B. (2014). Want to ace that test? Get the right kind of sleep. *The New York Times*. Retrieved from http://getcollegecredit.com/blog/article/8_tips_to_help_you_pass_a_standardized_test

Grohol, J. (2006). 10 highly effective study habits. Psych Central. Retrieved from http://psychcentral.com/lib/top-10-most-effective-study-habits/000599

Harris Health System. (2015). Forget all-night studying, a good night's sleep is key to doing well on exams. Retrieved from https://www.harrishealth.org/en/news/pages/sleep-key-doing-well-exams.aspx

National Council of State Boards of Nursing (NCSBN). (2012). Report of findings from the 2011 RN practice analysis: Linking the NCLEX-RN examination to practice. Chicago, IL: Author.

National Council of State Boards of Nursing (NCSBN). (2014a). NCSBN home page. Retrieved from https://www.ncsbn.org/index.htm

National Council of State Boards of Nursing (NCSBN). (2014b). Frequently asked questions. Retrieved from https://www.ncsbn.org/nclex-faqs.htm

National Council of State Boards of Nursing, National Council Licensure Examination for Registered Nurses (NCLEX-RN, 2012). NCLEX-RN test plan. Retrieved from https://www.ncsbn.org/2013_NCLEX_RN_Test_Plan.pdf

Prometric. (2014). 8 tips to help you pass a standardized test. Retrieved from http://getcollegecredit.com/blog/article/8_tips_to_help_you_pass_a_standardized_test

Russell, K. A. (2012). Nurse practice acts guide and govern nursing practice. *Journal of Nursing Regulation, 3*(3), 36–42.

Scholastic. (2015). It's brain food! Retrieved from http://www.scholastic.com/parents/resources/article/health-nutrition/its-brain-food

3

THE ROLE OF THE REGISTERED NURSE

ELEMENTS OF THE ROLE OF THE REGISTERED NURSE

1. Discusses being a professional

2. Examines professional practice and involvement

3. Defines autonomy and control over practice

4. Acknowledges the role of professional associations in professional development

5. Outlines the role of LPN/LVN

When you decided to become a registered nurse (RN), you probably had an accurate idea of what someone in the RN role does from a technical perspective. The technical perspective is easy to define: Pass medications, start an IV, carry out provider orders, and perform other physical and emotional aspects of caring for a patient. But you may not have thought about the professional aspects of the profession, nor about what a true profession entails. The first two chapters of this book discussed the definition and your legal scope of practice. This chapter will continue to build on your understanding of the RN role by focusing specifically on the professional role.

What Is a Professional, and Why Should You Care?

The word *profession* is used liberally, in many cases, in lieu of the word *job*. Many people consider their role in their job as their profession. However, the word *profession* has a distinct meaning, and it has criteria. All too often, nurses—whether early in their careers or seasoned—tend to think of their roles in a technical-job-oriented manner. In a time of immense change in healthcare, a time when many nurses long to spend more time with their patients, we want to demonstrate the value of what a nurse is meant to be—a professional with technical responsibilities.

A true profession has, at minimum, these elements:

- A unique body of knowledge
- A code of ethics
- Autonomy
- Academic education and preparation
- Self-regulation

QUESTIONS TO CONSIDER

1. What other professions exist?

2. Why must a profession have these standards?

3. What would nursing look like if it were not a profession?

4. Can a profession lose its "profession" status?

5. What is your responsibility as an RN in maintaining the professional standards?

6. How will you be involved in *your* profession so that nursing will continue to be a strong and trusted profession?

Many definitions of *profession* include additional elements, but whichever definition is used, nursing is considered a profession, one like law, medicine, and divinity. Nursing has a unique body of knowledge, separate from medicine. You can earn a PhD in nursing. This degree is a reflection of the research and theory that are unique to the nursing profession. The nursing code of ethics is maintained and updated regularly by the American Nurses Association (ANA).

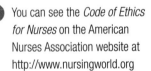 You can see the *Code of Ethics for Nurses* on the American Nurses Association website at http://www.nursingworld.org

Nursing education is also standardized by way of accreditation processes. Nursing schools are accredited by either the National League for Nursing (NLN) or the American Association of Colleges of Nursing (AACN). Both organizations provide standardized criteria by which undergraduate education is developed and taught.

Nursing is also a self-regulated profession. In the early 1900s, nurses sought to achieve a standard for nurses' education and practice. This effort included the creation of state boards of nursing in every state as the way to maintain the highest levels of practice in nursing, control over nursing education, and disciplinary processes for those who do not meet these standards. This level of self-regulation is granted by every state's legislature. By carrying out this self-regulation, the profession of nursing serves and maintains its service to the public.

As an RN, you are not part of the medical field. You are in the nursing profession, which is part of the *healthcare* field. By saying that you are part of the medical field, you are denouncing the body of nursing knowledge and saying, in effect, that nursing is not its own profession. Every time I hear a nurse say he or she is in the medical profession, it's like scraping fingernails on a chalkboard to me. Acknowledge that you are an RN, that nursing is a profession, and that you practice in the field of nursing.

DID YOU KNOW?

Nursing has been rated number-one on the Gallup Poll of Most Trusted Professions every year but one since it was first listed in 1999. (The exception was in 2001, when firefighters were voted number-one after the events of 9/11.) Can you imagine a time when the public wouldn't vote for nurses as the most trusted profession? We believe that nurses' high commitment to professional standards is one reason that the public trusts them. As you begin your journey into your nursing career, how will you continue to contribute to nursing's high professional standards?

Professional Practice

As a registered nurse, it is your responsibility to represent nursing in a professional manner. Nursing is not a job where you leave the workplace and leave your identity there, too. Your position as an RN with your employer will have boundaries, such as the times and dates you go to work, that separate your personal life from your work life. But you are an RN every day; every single hour of every single day, you represent nursing—and your fellow nurses. And this concept doesn't end when you clock out at the end of your shift. When you completed the NCLEX exam to become an

RN, you agreed to the rules and regulations of your state nurse practice act. That piece of paper with your RN license number on it allows you to practice as an RN as long as you follow your scope of practice. We encourage you to read your state nurse practice act and all updates published by your state board of nursing (BON).

Professional Involvement

Many nursing organizations are involved with different aspects of evolving the profession. These organizations include employed individuals and many RN volunteers. You can find a host of professional and specialty organizations with a variety of mission statements to join and belong to, and you can volunteer your time after you get started in your new career.

It is your professional responsibility to belong to professional and specialty organizations, such as the American Nurses Association (ANA) and Sigma Theta Tau International (STTI). You will need to make choices such as which ones to pay dues to and which ones to volunteer your time to. Paying dues to associations without volunteering your time is always acceptable, by the way. Doing the work of nursing requires money—thus, the term *pay to play.* For nursing organizations to be able to participate on state and national panels, they are expected to pay for seats at the table. Though these seats are expensive, they are worth every dollar to ensure that nursing's voice is heard. Consider this: If every nurse in the United States were to donate to the ANA political action committee (PAC), nurses as a united group would be one of the most powerful lobbying groups in Washington, DC.

Clinical Autonomy and Control Over Practice

At the base of professional practice are the terms *clinical autonomy* and *control over practice.* Autonomy is one of the original 14 forces of magnetism (McClure, Poulin, Sovie, & Wandelt, 1983), which is the original research, published in 1983, regarding Magnet hospitals. These two terms refer to the freedom, power, and authority to make decisions related to professional nursing practice; these terms, however, have subtle differences between them (Weston, 2009):

- **Clinical autonomy**—The authority, freedom, and discretion of nurses to indicate clinical nursing judgments concerning the care of individual patients (Weston, 2008).

- **Control over practice**—The authority, freedom, and discretion of nurses to make decisions related to the context of nursing practice, which includes organizational structures, governance, rules, policies, and operations (Weston, 2008).

These two terms are important in relation to the next section. As mentioned, these two terms are foundational to RN practice. Quite often, RNs do not view their practices as independent and do not view themselves as having clinical autonomy or control over their practices. But you do. This is not just for advanced practice registered nurses (APRNs). As an RN, you have your own scope, your own license, independent of and separate from the medical field. Though you may do some tasks based on physician orders, you do not report to physicians, nor is your practice under their purview.

ANA Standards of Practice and Professional Performance

Though every state board of nursing has its own legal scope of practice, the American Nurses Association also maintains the overarching scope for all RN practice. In many instances, state boards of nursing adopt this scope in their rules and regulations. Table 3.1 describes the ANA Standards of Nursing Practice and Professional Performance (ANA, 2010). These standards are broken out into two sections:

- **Practice**—Standards that apply to all RNs and APRNs; only standard 5D relates only to APRN practice.

- **Professional performance**—Standards that are not directly related to patient care but that are key aspects of the professional role.

Table 3.1   ANA Standards of Nursing Practice and Professional Performance

Standards of Practice	Standards of Professional Performance
Standard 1. Assessment	Standard 7. Ethics
Standard 2. Diagnosis	Standard 8. Education
Standard 3. Outcomes Identification	Standard 9. Evidence-Based Practice and Research
Standard 4. Planning	
Standard 5. Implementation	Standard 10. Quality of Practice
Standard 5A. Coordination of Care	Standard 11. Communication
Standard 5B. Health Teaching and Health Promotion	Standard 12. Leadership
	Standard 13. Collaboration
Standard 5C. Consultation	Standard 14. Professional Practice Evaluation
Standard 5D. Prescriptive Authority and Treatment	
	Standard 15. Resource Utilization
Standard 6. Evaluation	Standard 16. Environmental Health

(ANA, 2010)

Though we've given you only a snippet of information about your nursing scope, we recommend that you familiarize yourself with this topic in detail.

Specialty Standards of Practice

In many instances, in partnership with the American Nurses Association (ANA), specialty organizations have published specialty-specific standards of practices. Examples of specialty areas are addictions nursing, cardiovascular nursing, faith community nursing, forensic nursing, and home health nursing—and many, many more exist. In some instances, specialty standards are written collaboratively with other specialty nursing organizations. The nearby sidebar lists a few of the specialty nursing organizations.

EXPERIENCE FROM THE FIELD: THE GREAT NURSING ENDOWMENT

Like most other nurses, I usually make a quick stop for a helping of caffeine before the start of my shift. I used to never drink coffee. Never. In fact, I had proudly fought the need for this dangerous catalyst for a long time, until I eventually succumbed after a few years. Maybe it is because I work nights on a neuro floor, or maybe it's because it's just so hard to sleep during the day. If you have ever worked nights, you know exactly what I am talking about. It can be so challenging to get good sleep during the day. Your slumber is almost always interrupted by something simple, like your mother calling in the middle of the day and asking you some silly question or the awful sound of the trimmers and blowers from the landscapers. It's just enough sometimes to make you want to throw your phone out the window and yell out to the landscapers to hurry up.

Though many night nurses go to extremes to try to get good sleep by sleeping in their closets or investing in fancy noise and light reducers, I have chosen the simple solution. To me, building a soundproof section of my closet sounds not only completely unappealing but also like too much work in an attempt to sleep in less than desirable quarters. So I just stick with a little caffeine—plain and simple.

Most often, I find myself going through the drive-through before work. As I place my order, my mind usually wanders, just imagining what the baristas are thinking when I pull up to the window. Surely they must remember me. I always order the same thing: a chai tea latte and a blueberry muffin (that is, if one is available at 6:30 at night). I pull up around the same time every day, wearing the same blue uniform and, most often, remnants of the sleepy eyes that the baristas are used to seeing early in the morning. I despise that feeling because it makes me feel lazy for sleeping during the day.

So with a bit of shame at the thought of daytime sleeping, I round the corner and wonder whether today will be the day that I pull up to the window and hear the barista tell me that the person in front of me has paid for my drink. I mean, it could happen, right? We have all seen those news stories of someone paying for the person in line behind him, and then that same gesture of thoughtfulness continuing for the rest of the day. To be honest, it's not like I need, for financial reasons, someone to buy my coffee. If that were the case, I would never place an order to begin with. It's just that the simple notion of a stranger doing something kind at the start of my day is meaningful.

And that brings me to nursing. It is not easy being a floor nurse. The job has a tendency to be both physically and emotionally overwhelming, at the very least. For a nurse, the kindness of a genuine smile or another small gesture goes a long way. Nurses give so much to their patients and their families, but at the end of the day, what about us? Not to say that all the pizzas, cookie trays, and homemade treats brought in by families and patients don't count, but how do nurses support one another, and are we doing enough of it?

This question leads me to question the very heart and soul of our profession. Nursing theorist Jean Watson has stated that "caring is the essence of nursing." Not all nurses have had the honor to meet her, but they all have certainly heard of her, read about her, or at least learned about her pioneering work in a nursing theory class. This beautiful woman has dedicated her entire life and career to demonstrate and encourage the use of caring principles in healing because it is an essential part of our work.

Which brings me to my next point: If caring and compassion can assist in healing the wounded, can they not be used to heal our profession, which is plagued by evils such as lateral violence, apathy, and lack of involvement? Before evaluating this question, let's start from the beginning. If you were to take a moment to reflect on your nursing career, what impression would first come to mind? Would you recall a pivotal patient experience that has been gently tucked away in a corner of your heart? Will you feel an overwhelming sense of pride in knowing that patient care has improved in one way or another because of research you were involved in? Perhaps you will remember the profound influence that another nurse has had on you. Or maybe you are one of the many in the profession who now feels little other than indifference. Maybe you are simply too tired of caring for others and not being cared for enough in return.

It would not be unreasonable to think that, after all those years of opening your heart and sharing difficult times with your patients, you have turned down a bit of your humanity for self-preservation. For me, when I reflect on my career, all I can see are faces. They are the faces of accomplished nurse leaders who have been part of my journey since my time as a student nurse. They are the faces of the nurses who have inspired me and opened my eyes to situations that most floor nurses may never have the opportunity to experience. They are the faces of the people who have always believed in me as a nurse, but even more so as a valuable person to the future of our profession. Whenever I think about my past or contemplate my future, the people behind these faces are always a part of it. Whether they realize it or not, a piece of each of them is in everything I do. I am one of the lucky ones: Only a handful of other nurses I have ever met have had such extraordinary mentors. It is a tragedy to think that so many others either never took the time to seek guidance from more tenured nurses or were never received well when they did. So why is mentorship so important in nursing?

With some degree of confidence, I can tell you that most nurses have had a running start to their careers in clinical practice. That is, after all, why most people choose to become nurses. Some people spend their entire lives dreaming of braving the chaos of the emergency room, and others cannot wait to cradle and care for the newborn babies in post-partum. Some thrive on the thought of the adrenaline of traumas rolling in the doors, and others prefer the complex care of patients in the intensive care unit. No matter in which area of clinical practice you began or which one you transitioned to, you know that clinical practice can be nothing short of a beast.

Taking care of people who require care can be exhausting, and even beginning to learn in any of these environments is challenging all on its own. This does not even include the layers of issues that arise from intraprofessional relationships, staffing that does not account for patient acuity, nurse turnover, budget issues, and the fact that you know you have to clock out by a certain time at the end of the shift but you missed your break and have been to the bathroom only once. Phew.

The first few years for new nurses are by far the most important years in their careers because they are the most vulnerable. This is where their environment shapes their attitudes and work ethics. The statistics of nurse dropout rates within the first few years speak for themselves. I can tell you that as a new nurse, I was subjected to violence from my coworkers. I had no outside training beyond the floor, and it felt like I was expected to know everything. There was a tremendous amount of pressure with few resources available to me. At the end of a rough day, I would drive home, and all I could think of were those amazing nurses who believed in me. So I continued to push forward. I worked hard and began to work, first as a preceptor and then as a charge nurse for my unit.

With the increasing responsibilities, I began to see the staff in a different light. Most important, I began to see myself in a different light. I realized that without changing anything about the structure of my responsibilities, I could significantly impact the staff. I made it a point to know the professional goals of my coworkers. I always felt that it was important to encourage them to continue their pursuit of education, or their involvement within the organization, or to support their lingering urge to become more involved in a professional organization. It would take only a minute or so of my time, but I wanted to offer any help possible, no matter how seemingly insignificant. I genuinely cared about the staff. Over time, I saw the team change. I no longer saw lateral violence on the floor, and they became more confident in their abilities. The team members cared about each other. Of course, every group has exceptions (or weeds, as you may say), but teamwork was how we survived, and I could not have been more proud. I believe that an intelligent and genuinely caring leader can completely change an entire workplace environment. I have seen it happen. Most importantly, a great working environment translates to great patient care.

The point I want to make is that you should never underestimate the transformative power you hold. For me, just knowing that I had people to support me and help me grow has made all the difference. That is all you need to do. You can't do it for everyone, but you can start with only one bright-eyed coworker or a new graduate nurse on the floor and help that person not to become overwhelmed. If you can elicit a simple goal from her and help her seek opportunities to realize that goal, I can promise you a tenfold reward. It may not happen in a day, such as in the line for coffee where every customer buys a drink for the next customer in line. It may not even happen in a month. In fact, it may take years for your simple kindnesses to help other people grow in their careers, but maybe along the way, that person begins to help others, and then those others begin to help others, too. Kindness truly has powers beyond what we can even imagine. So that next time you reach for your coffee, just think about how you have the power to change your entire profession.

–Jasmine Bhatti, MSN, RN

The RN As a Leader

In Chapter 1, we introduced you to the report *The Future of Nursing* from the Institute of Medicine (IOM); in Chapter 6, we will go into depth about leadership. Another key recommendation from the IOM report is that RNs are prepared and enabled to lead change. Whether you want to be a leader or not, or whether you've even considered nurses as leaders, you *are* a leader. This concept might mean that you're leading and delegating to the care team on your unit or teaching health courses in your community or being a nurse on an organization's board of directors. The IOM recommendation specifically states:

> Recommendation 7: *Prepare and enable nurses to lead change to advance health.*
>
> *Nurses, nursing education programs, and nursing associations should prepare the nursing workforce to assume leadership positions across all levels, while public, private, and governmental health care decision makers should ensure that leadership positions are available to and filled by nurses (IOM, 2011, p. 14).*

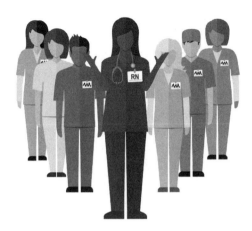

What Does This Mean for You?

Even if you think that you don't want to manage or to be a manager, that doesn't mean you are not a leader. Being a leader and being a manager are not synonymous. Many leaders are not formal managers, and everyone knows a manager who does not act like a leader. The healthcare system is an ever-changing environment. Nurses are at the front lines of care in all areas, and as part of the most trusted profession, nurses advocate for their patients and communities. As an RN, you are a leader, an advocate for everyone, and an advocate for healthcare. Let your voice be heard; let your experiences be known. Help make a positive impact in the healthcare system. All RNs are leaders. Lead from wherever you are. As author Tim Fargo says, "Leadership is service, not position."

The LPN Role in Healthcare

The licensed practical nurse (LPN) or licensed vocational nurse (LVN) has a valuable place in healthcare. The National League for Nursing (NLN) believes that licensed practical/vocational nurses are licensed professionals who are committed to providing safe quality care in a variety of healthcare environments (NLN, 2014).

According to the Bureau of Labor Statistics (2015), employment opportunities for LPNs/LVNs are projected to increase 22% by 2020. Though the employment opportunities are good, the practice settings have changed over the years from acute care to more long-term and outpatient settings (Health Resources and Services Administration [HRSA], 2013).

The LPN/LVN practices under a specific state license and nurse practice act, and most often under the direction of the registered nurse. Initially, LPNs/LVNs were trained to work in hospitals alongside registered nurses. LPNs now work in long-term care facilities, rehabilitation centers, schools, physician offices, clinics, correctional facilities, occupational organizations, mental health clinics, hospice care facilities, and home health agencies (Bureau of Labor Statistics, 2015; Practicalnursing.org, 2015).

All nurses should know and understand their role within the legal and healthcare systems. Working as a team, RNs and LPNs/LVNs must understand each role in order to provide safe, quality care. Shaffer, Johnson, and Guinn share that the LPN/LVN functions in a task-oriented role under the direction of the registered nurse, physician, or dentist, providing patient care and giving input into assessments, planning, and evaluating care while implementing the plan of care directed by the registered nurse (2010). Not surprisingly, Corazzini et al. (2011) found that 70% of the licensed care provided in long-term care facilities was given by LPN/LVN staff.

Individual state boards of nursing practice acts regulate the LPN/LVN scope of practice and how registered nurses direct the practice (NLN, 2014). Both RNs and LPNs/LVNs need to know and understand the scope of practice within the state where they are working. In addition, individual organizations may have limitations on the scope of practice for LPNs/LVNs. The NLN is sensitive to the fact that the LPN/LVN is an integral part of the broader scope of healthcare providers and is working to ensure that LPNs/LVNs receive adequate education to serve specific populations of patients and are not limited in the academic progression (NLN, 2014). The Bureau of Labor Statistics (2010–2011) provides detailed information on the responsibilities of the LPN in regards to providing direct patient care such as:

- Providing ongoing assessments

- Taking vital signs

- Bathing patients

- Feeding and toileting

- Administering medications

- Providing treatments

- Supervising nonlicensed staff

- Delegating

- Implementing emergency resuscitation procedures

> We will go into the ins and outs of delegation in Chapter 6.

- Contributing to the plan of care

- Supervising

Because nurses rarely work alone, you can expect to be working as a member of a team. Part of the team concept involves supervising others. You might supervise other registered nurses, licensed practical/vocational nurses, unlicensed staff, and students. Nurses are responsible for following the nurse practice act in the state in which they are licensed, the standards of practice, specific policies of the employing organization, and legal and ethical models of practice (Marthaler, 2003). Safe nursing practice requires good supervision.

QUESTIONS TO CONSIDER

1. How is the LPN/LVN legal scope of practice different from the RN scope of practice?

2. Have you read your state board of nursing's scope of practice, for not only RNs but also all nurses, LPNs/LVNs, and APRNs?

3. What effect will it have on your practice and your license if you do not know the legal scope of practice for those coworkers who are not RNs?

4. Have you looked at your state board of nursing's website for information on disciplinary processes?

5. Did you review those individuals who have had action taken against their license for practicing beyond their scope?

6. Would you know if you or a coworker were practicing outside of your legal scope?

As a professional, you will be held accountable for your scope of practice and standards of practice. It is important that you understand your legal and professional scope of practice. The RN plays an important role in the health of the nation, as not only clinicians but also leaders.

Chapter Checkup

Key points from this chapter include:

❑ All RNs are leaders!

❑ You have a professional scope of practice and professional standards of practice to which you will be held professionally accountable.

❑ You are a professional, so rather than say that you work somewhere, say that you practice instead: "I practice nursing in the medical surgical unit at . . . ."

❑ Belonging to professional nursing organizations and specialty nursing organizations is about more than paying for the dues. Paying dues is a minimum professional standard.

References

American Nurses Association (ANA). (2010). *Nursing: Scope and standards of practice* (2nd ed.). Silver Spring, MD: Nursing World.

Bureau of Labor Statistics, U.S. Department of Labor. (2015). *Occupational outlook handbook*, 2014–15 edition. Licensed practical and licensed vocational nurses. Retrieved from http://www.bls.gov/ooh/healthcare/licensed-practical-and-licensed-vocational-nurses.htm

Corazzini, K. N., Anderson, R. A., Mueller, C., McConnell, E. S., Landerman, L. R., Thorpe, J. M., & Short, N. M. (2011). Regulation of LPN scope of practice in long-term care. *Journal of Nursing Regulation, 2*(2), 30–36.

Health Resources and Services Administration (HRSA), Bureau of Health Professions. (2013). The U.S. nursing workforce: Trends in supply and education. Retrieved from http://bhpr.hrsa.gov/healthworkforce/supplydemand/nursing/nursingworkforce

Institute of Medicine (IOM). (2011). *The future of nursing: Leading change, advancing health*. Washington, DC: The National Academies Press.

Marthaler, M. (2003). Delegation of nursing care. In P. Kelly-Heidenthal (Ed.), *Nursing leadership and management* (pp. 266–279). Clifton Park, NY: Delmar.

McClure, M. L., Poulin, M. A, Sovie, M. D., & Wandelt, M. A. (1983). *Magnet hospitals: Attraction and retention of professional nurses*. Kansas City, MO: ANA.

National League of Nursing (NLN). (2014). A vision for recognition of the role of licensed practical/vocational nurses in advancing the nation's health. Retrieved from http://www.nln.org/docs/default-source/about/nln-vision-series-%28position-statements%29/nlnvision_7.pdf

Practicalnursing.org. (2015). 8 roles of the LPN. Retrieved from http://www.practicalnursing.org/8-roles-of-lpn

Shaffer, L. M., Johnson, K., & Guinn, C. (2010). Remedying role confusion: Differentiating RN and LPN roles. *American Nurse Today, 5*(3). Retrieved from http://www.americannursetoday.com/remedying-role-confusion-differentiating-rn-and-lpn-roles

Weston, M. J. (2008). Defining control over nursing practice and autonomy. *Journal of Nursing Administration, 38,* 404–408.

Weston, M. J. (2009). Validity of instruments for measuring autonomy and control over nursing practice. *Journal of Nursing Scholarship, 41*(1), 87–94. doi:10.1111/j.1547-5069.2009.01255.x

DEALING WITH LEGAL AND ETHICAL ISSUES

ELEMENTS OF DEALING WITH LEGAL AND ETHICAL ISSUES

1. Discusses working under legal and ethical codes

2. Defines key legal and ethical concepts

3. Provides ethical and legal case studies

4. Shows the Nightingale pledge

In this chapter, we will discuss the legal and ethical issues that nurses may encounter while working. Many of the legal and ethical terms and definitions that we will describe (some of which you may already know) will be helpful to you in carrying out your professional nurse duties. Nurses are confronted by ethical issues every day of their lives, and dealing with ethical issues as a professional may challenge a person's personal beliefs and moral structure. Nurses must also follow many types of laws and legal practices to maintain licensure and provide safe, quality care to patients.

Working Under Legal and Ethical Codes

As a nurse, you will be expected to understand the legal and ethical aspects of the professional nursing practice. If you were to fail to practice under moral, ethical, and legal codes, nothing would be in place to prevent harm to patients, families, and peers. The lists in this chapter identify some of the more common ethical and legal codes that nurses should understand and practice. In this chapter, we explore the different legal and ethical issues that nurses may encounter. Because we could not begin to explore every type of legal and ethical issue a nurse may face, we have chosen various case studies to explore together. We will begin by discussing the ethics related to the nursing profession.

You may work in patient care areas often in quite stressful situations that present different types of ethical scenarios. Frequently, when people are placed in stressful situations, they react to decisions and circumstances differently than they normally would respond. Over time, nurses may be confronted by many ethical and moral issues that challenge their personal belief systems. Although morals and ethics are similar in that they relate to right and wrong, they are different by definition.

- *Morals* comprise an individual's belief system; specifically, they form an individual's "compass" to help distinguish right from wrong.

- *Ethics* are rules, or guidelines, to help distinguish right from wrong. They are provided by an outside source or professional entity.

Nurses practice under a general code of ethics, which is a guideline for working with patients, peers, healthcare professionals, and the general public. The first known nursing code of ethics was the *Nightingale pledge,* developed by Lystra Gretter, a nurse instructor. The Nightingale pledge was structured after the Hippocratic oath, which is taken by physicians (Gretter, 1910).

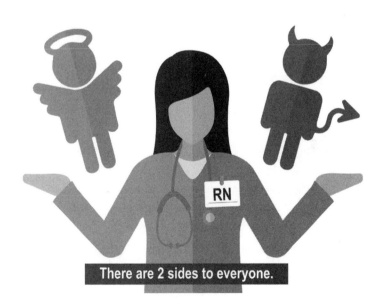

There are 2 sides to everyone.

Since that time, suggested and tentative ethical codes have been explored with several revisions to the original *Code for Professional Nurses* first introduced by the American Nurses Association (ANA) in 1950 (ANA, 1950). Subsequently, the code has been revised multiple times and now includes interpretive statements as a practice guide for professional nurses (ANA, 2008).

The American Nurses Association (ANA) *Code of Ethics for Nurses with Interpretive Statements* (the *Code of Ethics for Nurses*) explicates the goals, values, and ethical precepts that direct the profession of nursing. The ANA believes that the *Code of Ethics for Nurses* is nonnegotiable and that each nurse has an obligation to uphold and adhere to the code (ANA, 2015).

ETHICAL TERMS

There are many ethical situations that you as a nurse may find yourself in as you progress in your career as a registered nurse (RN). As nurses, we must work within ethical boundaries to ensure that our patients, peers, and selves are provided and are giving quality care, patients are not mistreated, patients and nurses have a voice, and patients and nurses are treated with respect. It is very important to know and understand ethical terms that might be used in a court of law. These terms include *ethics, ethical dilemma, bioethics, fidelity, veracity, beneficence, non-maleficence, justice, morals, autonomy, values,* and *values clarification.*

- **Ethics**—The branch of philosophy that examines the differences between right and wrong
- **Ethical dilemma**—A conflict between two or more ethical principles
- **Bioethics**—The application of general ethical principles to health-care
- **Fidelity**—The ethical foundation of nurse–client relationships
- **Veracity**—Truthfulness; neither lying to nor deceiving others
- **Beneficence**—The duty to promote good and to prevent harm, including the two integral elements of providing benefit and balancing benefit and harm

- **Non-maleficence**—The duty to cause no harm to others
- **Justice**—The obligation to be fair
- **Morals**—The private, personal, or group standards of right and wrong
- **Autonomy**—The individual's right to choose and the ability to act on that choice
- **Value**—A belief you have about the worth of something; an ideal, a belief, a custom, a mode of conduct, a quality, or a goal that is highly prized or preferred by individuals, groups, or society; serves as a principle or standard that influences decision-making
- **Values clarification**—The analysis of one's own values to better understand what is truly important

(Marquis & Huston, 2015; Sullivan, 2013)

Seeing Nursing Ethics in Action: Case Studies

We have supplied the case studies in this chapter to show you the ways these ethical principles surround you and what you can do every day in your work environment and professional practice. You may identify with a specific case because you have witnessed it happening or you were in some way personally involved. When you read the case study, analyze the particular actions of the nurse, and consider what you personally would have done, should have done, or simply could not do. Each case is followed by an answer regarding the ethical principle in question.

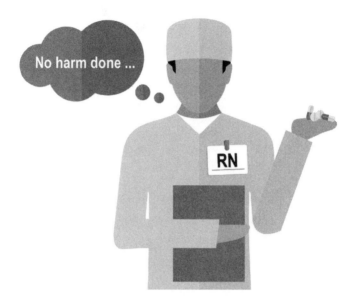

Beneficence

Ben, tired from working his fourth 12-hour overnight shift of the week on an unusually busy night, has prepared and administered 60 milligrams of Cardizem to one of his patients. The elderly patient questions the color of the pill, stating that he usually takes a green pill at home for his heart condition. Ben responds, "Now I'm the nurse, and I know I gave you the correct medication."

Later, when Ben checks the patient's medication orders, he discovers that the physician had decreased the Cardizem to 30 milligrams earlier in the shift. The new order had not been transcribed and sent to the pharmacy. Ben decides that no harm has been done to the patient and that no one will know about the error he has made, because the patient has been known to have periods of confusion.

Did Ben do anything wrong? Did he violate any ethical principles?

Answer

Ben violated several ethical principles. First, he violated the principle of beneficence, or doing no harm. By not stopping to recheck the medication, he gave the wrong dose to the patient. Ben also violated the patient's right to autonomy, because the patient questioned the medication. Ben also violated the principle of veracity, because he lied to himself by not self-reporting the medication error. Are there any other ethical and or legal principles violated?

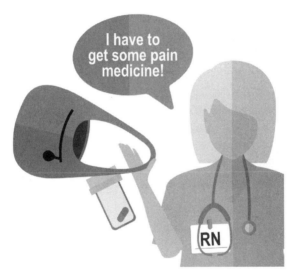

Stealing

Susie suffers from an unrelenting toothache during her shift. She checks her purse for aspirin but finds the container empty. She recalls, however, that there is stock ibuprofen in the medication room, so Susie takes four tablets to reduce the pain of her tooth-ache. The other nurses were in patient rooms and did not see Susie take the ibuprofen.

Did Susie violate any ethical principles?

Answer

Yes, Susie violated the principle of veracity by taking the ibuprofen. She also violated the principle of fidelity, because she violated the core of the the nurse–employee relationship. She may also become impaired since she took a large dose of the ibuprofen, placing not only herself, but the patients and the organization in for ethical and legal risks. What other ethical and or legal principles were violated?

A Difficult Decision?

Gene has been late for work several times over the past 2 months and was recently informed that he would be terminated if he were late again. As he drives to work one morning, suddenly a pedestrian is struck by a car ahead of Gene. The person is clearly injured, and the driver has failed to stop.

Gene has an ethical dilemma: Continue on to work to avoid being late and subsequently losing his job, or stop and help the injured person, which would put his job status in jeopardy.

What would you do?

Answer

Sometimes, you must step up to help others in need even if you suffer a loss. Generally, no one will fault others for not putting themselves at risk for dying. However, always ask yourself whether you would want someone to help you if you were in a dire situation.

Autonomy

You are an RN employed in an emergency department (ED). One afternoon a 95-year old patient is admitted from a local long-term care facility and diagnosed with dehydration and a urinary tract infection. He also has a history of coronary artery disease. He is refusing to have an IV started for hydration and an IV antibiotic administered. As the nurse, you are aware that a failure to receive proper fluids and the prescribed medication may lead the patient toward confusion, severe dehydration, and possible cardiac and kidney failure. The physician has ordered you to start the IV anyway, in spite of the patient's refusal and his direct statement, "Just let me die. I want to go be with my wife."

What would you do? Do you assume that the patient is confused and making an irrational decision? Is the patient exercising any of his rights? Can the physician make you start the IV?

Answer

Patients have the right (of autonomy) to make their own, informed decisions about their care. As a nurse, you must always ensure that patients have sufficient information, including both positive and negative aspects, so that they can realistically make informed decisions. You must also consider whether patients are confused or unable to make informed decisions because of mental illness, dementia, or metabolic syndromes that might interfere with the ability to make sound decisions.

If you believe that a patient is unable to make an informed decision, it is appropriate to include any family members, persons holding power of attorney over healthcare needs, and case managers or social workers who may need to assist the patient legally.

In a situation where a patient is of sound mind and may make an informed decision, it is illegal and unethical to coerce the patient into accepting unwanted procedures, even if you do not agree with the decision.

As these case studies show, as an RN you need to be aware of the ethical issues surrounding the situations you will face. The ethical principles of the profession provide helpful guidelines to follow when your personal feelings or morals may pull you in another direction. The guidelines can ensure that you keep patients and their care foremost in your mind. If a situation requires making a decision about ethics and you are unsure what to do, organizations generally have good resource people who may be quite helpful, such as a chaplain or another member of the clergy, a member of the ethics committee, or the nurse manager or director.

Now turn your attention to legal matters that impact your nursing.

LEGAL TERMS

The legal terms in this sidebar are ones that nurses need to be familiar with to help protect themselves and their patients from suffering legal turmoil. RNs are privileged to be licensed, but that license comes with legal responsibilities. Healthcare is an extremely complex concept, with many legal issues that might arise while providing care to patients. It is not uncommon for patients and family members to ask the nurse for answers to their questions and even for advice. Maybe it has even happened to you. How did you respond? Did you place yourself in a potentially illegal position? Some of the more common terms we discuss are *do not resuscitate, negligence, unprofessional conduct, whistleblowing, advance directives, advance medical care directive, advocate, assault and battery, durable power of attorney, informed consent, invasion of privacy, living will, malpractice, false imprisonment,* and *falsification of records.*

- **Advance directive**—Written instructions that are recognized under state law and related to the provision of such care when the individual is capacitated
- **Advance medical care directive**—A document in which the individual, in consultation with the physician, relatives, or other personal advisers, provides precise instructions for the type of care the client wants in specific situations
- **Advocate**—A person who speaks up for or acts on behalf of the client
- **Assault**—The act of threatening bodily harm to a patient
- **Battery**—A violent act committed on a patient with the intent to cause harm

- **Do not resuscitate**—An order, written by the physician, that provides an exception to the universal standing order to resuscitate or perform other lifesaving measures on the patient

- **Durable power of attorney (healthcare proxy)**—An authorization that enables any competent individual to name someone to exercise decision-making authority, under specific circumstances, on the individual's behalf

- **False imprisonment**—To restrain a patient in an area without justification or consent

- **Falsification of records**—The intentional alteration or fabrication of any information on the client record

- **Informed consent**—A person's agreement to allow something to happen based on the full disclosure of facts needed to make an intelligent decision. The agreement must include information about the procedure or treatment and why it is needed, the risks involved, its benefits, any alternative-treatment options, and the consequences of refusal. Informed consent is required for surgery, certain diagnostic and medical treatments, and research involving clients

- **Invasion of privacy**—An unwanted intrusion of a client's personal affairs

- **Living will**—A document prepared by a competent adult that provides direction regarding medical care in the event the person becomes unable to make decisions personally

- **Malpractice**—Negligence committed by a professional, such as a nurse or physician, that produces harm to the client

- **Negligence**—Conduct that falls below the professional standard of care. An example is the act of doing something that a reasonable and prudent nurse would not do

- **Unprofessional conduct**—Conduct that could adversely affect the health and welfare of the public

- **Whistleblowing**—Reporting conduct that is incompetent, illegal, or unethical

(Marquis & Huston, 2015; Miller, 2015; Sullivan, 2013)

Seeing Nursing Legal Issues in Action: Case Studies

We have created the following case studies to show you the ways these legal principles affect you and what you do every day in your work environment and professional practice. You may have already experienced a similar situation or have witnessed one, but did you think about the legal issues that might arise as a result of your actions or lack of action? The following case studies are presented for you to carefully consider what actions or lack of action could lead to future legal problems. Each case is followed by an answer that reflects the legal principle that was violated.

Code or No Code

You enter a patient's room and find the patient to be in full respiratory arrest. You start CPR and call for the code team. When the code team arrives, one nurse states that the patient is documented to be a no-code.

Do you stop the resuscitation efforts? Are legal issues in effect because a code was started in spite of the no-code documentation?

Answer

Yes, you may stop the resuscitation measures if you have clear and accurate documentation that the person has declared that no heroic measures are to be taken when a life-threatening event occurs. Ceasing your lifesaving efforts may be difficult when the event is already taking place, and nurses and physicians may then be reluctant to stop their resuscitation measures for fear of being sued by the patient, if he or she survives, or family. However, the law provides protection if the patient has expressed resuscitation desires in writing.

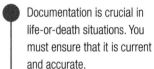 Documentation is crucial in life-or-death situations. You must ensure that it is current and accurate.

Patient Abuse?

A nurse tech has reported to the charge nurse that Mr. Cook, a confused patient, hit her in the stomach when she attempted to lift him to the chair. When the charge nurse asks how the nurse tech handled the situation, the tech states, "I hit him back. He had no right to hit me." When the charge nurse assesses the patient, she finds a large, discolored area on the patient's right arm.

What legal issues may be identified? Did the nurse tech violate any legal or ethical issues? How should the charge nurse deal with the situation?

Answer

The nurse tech committed patient abuse (assault) by striking the patient. Even if a patient may strike out at you, it is generally understood that the person may be under stress or suffering from medication side effects or may have confusion or dementia. Though it is never acceptable for patients to strike or abuse nurses or any other healthcare providers, neither is it acceptable for nurses or healthcare providers to strike patients unless they experience a real or perceived threat of bodily harm.

In this situation, the patient (or the patient's family) legally has the right to file a lawsuit against the nurse tech and the hospital for patient abuse. In determining whether the case is valid, questions may be asked such as whether there was a foreseeable risk of harm or whether the patient is mentally competent.

A number of the sources in the "References" section of this chapter, including the ANA *Code of Ethics for Nurses with Interpretive Statements* and Miller's Legal/Ethical Terms in Nursing flash cards, make good sources to brush up on the legal and ethical terms we discuss in this chapter.

Nurses are taught techniques and communication strategies to defuse or avoid the risk of being harmed. We are not indicating that nurses or healthcare providers may not defend themselves in the event of being confronted with a real threat of danger. Nurses and other care providers may also be assault victims and may have the right to initiate legal action against the person. You should take every measure to defuse a situation so that no one gets hurt.

Invasion of Privacy

A nurse is asked by a friend to check on her friend's mother to see whether the laboratory has returned its pathology report. The nurse enters the organization's online computer program and finds the patient's pathology report, and then reads it and sends the results to her friend via text message.

What legal issues are identified? How would you handle this situation if you were being asked to seek medical information for your friend or if you witnessed another nurse do it?

Answer
The nurse violated several legal and ethical principles. Friends may mean well and have the best intentions, but it is unlawful and violates privacy laws (such as HIPAA) when a nurse, or any other care provider, seeks information about a patient for whom the nurse is not directly providing care. The nurse violated privacy laws when texting the information to her friend without the consent of the patient. She also engaged in unprofessional behavior and was negligent, because the action was considered not what a prudent nurse would do. The nurse also violated nursing ethics, morals, fidelity (truthfulness), veracity (the foundation of the nurse–patient relationship), and autonomy (the patient's right to decide to release the information). In many organizations, the nurse's employment would be terminated and she would have to

appear before the state board of nursing (BON) for the potential loss of or suspension of her license.

Informed Consent

As the nurse is preparing the patient for transport to surgery, the patient states that he is unsure what to expect will happen during the surgery. The nurse checks the signed informed consent on the patient's chart and tells the patient that he has already signed the form and that his surgeon does not like to be delayed.

What legal issues did the nurse violate? What would you have done in this situation?

Answer

The patient has the right to be fully informed of any procedure that he will experience. The nurse violated the right to an informed consent by not asking the patient whether the surgeon has fully explained the upcoming surgery and by not having the patient explain in his own words what the surgery will entail. The surgeon must explain fully and in language that the patient understands before the patient signs the informed consent and begins the procedure. The nurse must act as a patient advocate and not be negligent while doing everything possible to ensure that the patient is fully informed. The nurse in this case study should contact the surgeon and explain that the patient is unsure about the details of the surgery, inform the receiving nurse of the issue, and, if necessary, postpone the surgery if the patient is not fully informed.

The Nightingale Pledge

I solemnly pledge myself before God and in the presence of this assembly, to pass my life in purity and to practice my profession faithfully. I will abstain from whatever is deleterious and mischievous, and will not take or knowingly administer any harmful drug. I will do all in my power to maintain and elevate the standard of my profession, and will hold in confidence all personal matters committed to my keeping and all family affairs coming to my knowledge in the practice of my calling. With loyalty will I endeavor to aid the physician in his work, and devote myself to the welfare of those committed to my care (Gretter, 1893).

Registered nurses are consistently considered to be trustworthy by their patients. To maintain that trustworthiness, nurses must work within a framework of ethical and legal principles. These principles help to guide the nurse's decision-making process and ensure that patients are given safe, quality, ethical care. Nurses must also support their peers to ensure that everyone is given the respect due to their position. Nurses must uphold the ethical and legal practice of the registered nurse, supported by the nursing credentialing organizations, such as the American Nurses Association, the American Association of Colleges of Nursing (AACN), and the individual state boards of nursing (BON) that regulate nursing practice, state by state. We have provided in this chapter many definitions of ethical and legal principles and case studies to demonstrate how these principles may be violated. Carefully and periodically review these principles to ensure that you are engaged in safe, ethical, and legal practice and will not risk losing your nursing license.

Chapter Checkup

Key points from this chapter include:

❏ You must work within legal, ethical, and moral codes.

❏ You must know your own moral and ethical boundaries.

❏ Your moral and ethical boundaries may be challenged.

❏ You must uphold the legalities of the professional nurse practice.

❏ You have a responsibility to patients in your care but also to yourself and your peers.

References

American Nurses Association (ANA). (1950). ANA *House of Delegates Proceedings, Vol. I.* New York, NY: ANA.

American Nurses Association (ANA). (2008). *Guide to the code of ethics for nurses: Interpretation and application.* Silver Spring, MD: ANA.

American Nurses Association (ANA). (2015). Code of ethics for nurses with interpretive statements. Retrieved from http://www.nursingworld.org/MainMenuCategories/EthicsStandards/CodeofEthicsforNurses/Code-of-Ethics-For-Nurses.html

Gretter, L. (1910). Florence Nightingale pledge: Autographed manuscript dated 1893. *American Journal of Nursing 10*(4), 271.

Marquis, B. L., & Huston, C. J. (2015). *Leadership roles and management functions in nursing: Theory and application* (8th ed.). Philadelphia, PA: Wolters Kluwer Health.

Miller, L. A. (2015). Legal/ethical terms in nursing. Flash cards. Retrieved from https://quizlet.com/9259944/legalethical-terms-in-nursing-flash-cards

Sullivan, E. J. (2013). *Effective leadership and management in nursing* (8th ed.). Upper Saddle River, NJ: Pearson Education.

5

WORKING IN TEAMS

ELEMENTS OF WORKING IN TEAMS

1. Examines working as a team

2. Considers the RN role as a leader

3. Understands the importance of being trans-disciplinary

4. Discusses creating a highly effective team

5. Reflects on personal experiences

As a registered nurse (RN), you will always work in some sort of team arrangement to take care of patients. Healthcare teams are vital in achieving excellent patient care. Each person contributes in some way to patient care because no lone person can do it all, and should not try. You should understand some basic concepts about teamwork, the larger team, and your role on the healthcare team. This chapter will discuss your role as a team member, your role as the care coordinator, different members of the team, and vital tips for developing high-functioning teams.

Being a Good Team Member

An important first step in working on a team is to know how to be an effective team member. We don't mean that you should volunteer to do everything, however. Care delivery does not happen with nurses only; nurses and patients rely on a team of professionals to help deliver that care (Mensik, 2013). Therefore, all team members must:

- Understand the scope and role of all individuals who may care for patients.

- Ensure that the nursing staff understands the roles and delineates roles for everyone.

- Utilize other disciplines to their full potential, ability, and scope to provide patient care.

- Understand that RNs do not need to provide all aspects of a patient's care (Anderson et al., 2014).

The teams you will be on will vary in scope, from the care team for a group of patients to a shared governance team or a hospital initiative team. Despite the diversity of members or scope, this information is applicable at all levels.

You're the Team Leader/Care Coordinator

As a new RN, you are already a leader. You are also a care coordinator. This *is* the role of the RN, not just certain RNs in offices or case management. The care coordination is an essential part of all registered nurses' practice, and one standard of professional practice for nurses (ANA, 2010). Care coordination is "(a) a function that helps ensure that the patient's needs and preferences are met over time with respect to health services and information sharing across people, functions, and sites; and (b) the deliberate organization of patient care activities between two or more participants (including the patient) involved in a patient's care to facilitate the appropriate delivery of health care services" (ANA, 2012, p. 1).

 DID YOU KNOW?

RNs and advanced practice registered nurses (APRNs) have been performing care coordination as a core part of the nursing discipline since the early 20th century (ANA, 2012).

The lack of effective care coordination results in increased cost, potential adverse drug interactions, increased medical error, and unnecessary duplication of tests and services (IOM, 2003).

The targeting of team-based care—matching resources to patient and family needs (Anderson et al., 2014) where the RN acts as the care coordinator—leads to effective care coordination. The incorporation of multiple perspectives in healthcare offers the benefit of diverse knowledge and experience (Mitchell, 2012).

Improving Outcomes with Care Coordination

Research reported by the American Nurses Association shows that when nursing is involved in care coordination, outcomes across the board improve, including these benefits:

- Reductions in emergency department visits
- Noticeable decreases in medication costs
- Reduced inpatient charges
- Reduced overall charges
- Average savings per patient
- Significant increases in survival with fewer readmissions
- Lower total annual Medicare costs for those beneficiaries participating in pilot projects compared to control groups
- Increased patient confidence in self-managing care
- Improved quality of care
- Increased safety of older adults during transition from acute care settings to the home
- Improved clinical outcomes and reduced costs
- Improved patient satisfaction overall (ANA, 2012)

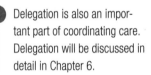 Delegation is also an important part of coordinating care. Delegation will be discussed in detail in Chapter 6.

However, to achieve these outcomes, an RN must be an effective team leader in the role of care coordinator.

Despite the length of time nurses may have been in leadership roles, they all must continue to learn more about leadership, and about themselves as leaders. Table 5.1 provides tips for new team leaders; however, these are helpful reminders for even the most seasoned of leaders.

Table 5.1   Tips for New Team Leaders

Tip	Why?
Overcommunicate	Be open and transparent. People who don't know you may be nervous to ask. Even if you don't know an answer, just say so. Do not think that you need to know everything— you will not and you cannot.
Ask questions	Many times, as a leader, you are expected to know. Shift your impression of yourself from "knower" to "learner." Spend half your time learning and asking questions of the team, not simply telling them what needs to be done.
Figure out what people truly want to do	Get to know the members of your team. Understand what they are most excited about. Accomplishments are common when the right person is filling the right role.
Get your hands dirty	Regardless of your role or position, spend some time doing the work of your team. This strategy helps give you a perspective that you might have lost, or that you never had in the first place.
Be decisive	Make decisions. The longer it takes for a decision to be made, the more unrest the team has as they struggle to function in uncertainty.

(DeWitt, 2014)

Though it may seem that Table 5.1 is simply a list of tips to run a meeting, our suggestions are applicable in your work with patients and their families. You may need to coordinate a patient/family care coordination meeting on the unit for a complex patient. The tips in Table 5.1 can help you become more effective for any type of meeting you will encounter.

Types of Teams in Healthcare

As mentioned previously, teams in healthcare may range from department-based with only clinicians and employees to a care coordination meeting with the patient, the patient's family members, and various clinicians. For now, we will focus on those teams providing healthcare services. *Team-based healthcare* is the provision of health services to individuals, families, and/ or their communities by at least two health providers who work collaboratively with patients and their caregivers (Naylor & Sochalski, 2010). This format aims to accomplish shared goals within and across settings to achieve coordinated, high-quality care (Naylor & Sochalski, 2010). Many types of teams exist, such as interdisciplinary, interprofessional, and transdisciplinary. All these terms partially refer to the composition of the members. Often these terms are used interchangeably; however, they are unique.

Consider these definitions:

- **Interdisciplinary/interprofessional team**—Teamwork within and across settings, in an effort to integrate and coordinate care

- **Intradisciplinary team**—Teamwork within a single profession, such as a team of nurses

- **Transdisciplinary team**—Transformation of your practice as you remain aware of how all other disciplines practice individually so that you can function to the highest extent in your role with the other team members in providing care to the user (Anderson et al., 2014, p. 29)

Each of these team types has a purpose and fits a specific need. For instance, if you are working on a unit-based nursing practice policy, you may have a team that is purely intradisciplinary. The goal of the project should guide the type of team you need. Remember to think outside the box, or outside the nursing box.

EXPERIENCE FROM THE FIELD: TEAMWORK

As you start your nursing career, your mind is full of new knowledge. The good news about being a good team member is that the strategies are the same in the workplace as they are outside the workplace. You probably already know how to be a team player. Now you just need to practice good teamwork every day.

There is one major difference that comes with teamwork in healthcare, as opposed to that in other professions. The difference is what is at stake if you do not have a high-functioning team. If you are playing a ballgame and not working as a team, the worst thing that can happen is that you might lose the game. If you are not working as a team in healthcare, people can get hurt or, even worse, lose their lives. Because the stakes are high, there is no room for a poor team player in nursing and healthcare.

First, look in the mirror. Are you a good team player? Do you speak directly to your coworkers when you have a concern? Do you avoid talking about your colleagues? If you overhear someone else speaking negatively about a team member, do you tell the person that it's inappropriate to talk about others and request that the concern be directed to the person involved?

Do you trust your team, and can you be trusted? Can you forgive? Everyone makes mistakes, and you need to be able to forgive in order to grow. Do you appreciate every team member's contribution to your work?

If you answered no to any of these questions, first work on your own behaviors. It's difficult to be a poor team member when you're surrounded by good team members, so you need to do your part.

There is nothing like having to float that brings out a nurse's true colors. Think about a time when a team member had to float to another unit. Was the floating nurse gracious, and did he have a positive attitude? Did the person make positive statements such as, "Oh, floating is fine. They always treat me so nicely," or toxic-sounding statements such as, "I hate that place. They always dump on me"? A nurse with toxic sentiment might grumble under his breath, question another unit's needs and motivations, and intentionally grab a cup of coffee on the way to the other unit so that he arrives late. Toxic behaviors can be overt or passive-aggressive. Neither is okay.

Lastly, as you think about teamwork, contemplate why you went into nursing. It's about the patient. If you keep the patient at the center of all that you do in your nursing career, you will be able to let go of small differences with team members. When you think about the patient at the end of her life, the new mom, the toddler with a new cancer diagnosis, or any other patient, you will want to be the best nurse on the best team so that the patient has every opportunity to have a positive experience.

–Deb Compton, MSN, RN, CCRN

Transdisciplinary Team as a Preferred Team Approach

Every team leader may build team membership for different reasons. The reasons may be based on specific needs, the number of people available, or deadlines, for example. Though each team type serves a specific person, care coordination specifically is best done by using a transdisciplinary team approach. As the RN, when you understand the roles and skills of all team members, you can delegate effectively. Additionally, the right person does the right thing at the right time. RNs do not need to perform all aspects of a patient's care.

However, the failure of RNs to delegate appropriately, or even not at all, because they don't know their team members or their scopes and abilities can result in poor quality of care and the breakdown of the team. As the RN, you cannot provide all of the care, even in a total patient care nursing model. Approaching care coordination, or even unit-based projects, through a transdisciplinary lens will allow you to ensure that outcomes, including staff satisfaction for everyone, are met.

Characteristics of a Highly Functioning Team

As time passes, research and evidence on teams change and advance our knowledge of this social phenomenon. What social and organizational scientists thought comprised a good team a decade ago differs and evolves into what we have today, as much as science advances and we learn even more in the next decade. Regardless of the type of team you are on, similarities across any of them lead them to be highly functional teams. Table 5.2 lists the top five characteristics of a highly functional team.

Table 5.2   Characteristics of a Highly Effective Team

Characteristic	Why?
Trust	When individuals can say anything without fear of retribution, you will manage less and lead more. The team will accomplish much more than it would in an environment lacking trust.
Clarity	When individuals on a team know the mission and vision, actions and progression occur. If the team is unsure of the goal, you are expecting members to create an action plan that may not achieve the expected goal.
Enabled	Allow team members to make decisions and create an action plan. Empower them to make change. (Theme: The leader is not always, and should not always be, the one with all the answers. That is known as *micromanaging*.)
Celebration of milestones	Ensure that team members are acknowledged for the work they have accomplished, and celebrate milestones. The continuous pursuit of goals without recognition of achievements is demoralizing.

Spotting a Dysfunctional Team

Whether at work or school, many people have experienced a dysfunctional team, though they may not be sure of its characteristics.

Despite all the research on highly effective teams, watch out for characteristics that can pull a team into dysfunction. Table 5.3 describes characteristics to be aware of when working on a team that may be dysfunctional, with methods to course-correct.

Table 5.3 Characteristics of Dysfunctional Teams

Characteristic	How to Course-Correct
Lack of commitment	Have members write down a list of everything the team accomplished during the past year. Frequently, teamwork focuses on the issue or problem and does not celebrate success. If people feel that they are never achieving anything, they may feel undervalued and unmotivated to try. Note and celebrate accomplishments.
Absence of trust	Be as inclusive as you can. When planning or working on a task, especially when you think you have the correct solution, the exclusion will alienate others. Remember that people will not destroy that which they helped to create.
Avoidance of accountability	Examine limiting assumptions and attitudes and remove them. Discuss with the team the beliefs that are creating the current culture. Then, together, write a statement that reflects where the team wants to go. Also assign specific team members to goals and actions. Make individuals responsible rather than the team.
Fear of conflict	Develop a set of team standards that everyone agrees on. Let everyone be accountable for holding others responsible for meeting these standards. When you build trust, this fear will also decrease.
Inattention to results	Assign specific team members to goals and actions. Make an individual responsible, rather than the team, and have that person report the results.

(Kent, 2009)

REFLECTING ON YOUR TEAM EXPERIENCES

Reflect freely on any type of experience, good or bad. You can learn from good experiences, and you can learn (such as what not to do) from the bad.

Think back to a time when you were on a highly functioning team:

1. What did the leader do to make the team highly functional?

2. How did you feel working on this team?

3. How did the team work together?

4. What is one thing you learned from this team that you will use as a leader on future teamwork?

Think back to a time when you were on a dysfunctional team:

1. What did the leader do or allow that made the team dysfunctional?

2. How did you feel working on this team?

3. How well did the team work together?

4. What is one thing you learned from this team that you will use as a leader on future teamwork?

Fostering Teamwork in a Negative Work Culture

Overall organizational or unit culture can have a negative effect on leading, and on teamwork. One unique approach to addressing a negative culture is the Pickle Challenge, which is part of the Florence Challenge. The Pickle Challenge includes a pledge that staff members take: "Take every complaint and turn it into a blessing or a constructive suggestion." Pickle jars are placed on the unit. Every time someone breaks the pledge, that person has to place money into the jar. The unit then decides, before or after the jar is full, where to send the money, to either charity or team projects.

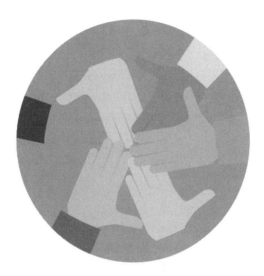

Earlier in this chapter, we talked about holding others accountable, creating trust, and developing commitment. This section has described another method to do that on your unit.

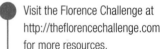
Visit the Florence Challenge at http://theflorencechallenge.com for more resources.

Effective team-building and effective leadership are skills that all RNs will continue to learn over their careers. In the beginning you will be a novice, but you will quickly learn and then build effective skills over your career. This strategy is the key to achieving excellent patient outcomes.

Chapter Checkup

Key points from this chapter include:

❑ Incorporate personal responsibility into being an excellent team member.

❑ As the RN, you are a care coordinator, and you are a leader.

❑ A lack of effective care coordination results in increased cost, potential drug interactions, increased medical error, and unnecessary duplication of tests and services.

❑ Thinking through a transdisciplinary lens transforms your practice because you are aware of how all other disciplines practice individually.

❑ Reflect and learn from good and bad teams. Both show you what to do and what not to do and are great learning experiences.

References

American Nurses Association (ANA). (2010). *Nursing: Scope and standards of practice* (2nd ed.). Silver Spring, MD: Nursing World.

American Nurses Association (ANA). (2012). *The value of nursing care coordination: A white paper of the American Nurses Association.* Silver Spring, MD: Nursing World.

Anderson, R., Ellerbe, S., Haas, S., Kerfoot, K., Kirby, K., & Nickitas, D. (2014). In J. Mensik (Ed.), *Excellence and evidence in staffing: A data-driven model for excellence in staffing* (2nd ed.). *Nursing Economic$, 32*(3 Suppl.), 1–36.

DeWitt, J. (2014). Leading teams: 5 tips for new team leaders. *Harvard Business Review.* Retrieved from https://hbr.org/2014/09/5-tips-for-new-team-leaders

Institute of Medicine (IOM). (2003). *Priority areas for national action: Transforming health care quality.* Washington, DC: The National Academies Press.

Kent, M. D. (2009). 5 dysfunctional traits of a team and 5 strategies to resolve them. *Hospital News and Healthcare Report, 5*(7). Retrieved from http://southfloridahospitalnews.com/page/5_Dysfunctional_Traits_of_a_Team_and_5_Strategies_to_Resolve_Them/3692/1/

Mensik, J. (2013). *The nurse manager's guide to innovative and effective staffing.* Indianapolis, IN: Sigma Theta Tau International.

Mitchell, P. M., Wynia, M., Golden, R., McNellis, B., Okun, S., Webb, C. E., ... Von Kohorn, I. (2012). *Core principles & values of effective team-based health care.* Washington, DC: Institute of Medicine.

Naylor, M. D., & Sochalski, J. A. (2010). Scaling up: Bringing the transitional care model into the mainstream. *Journal of Nursing Administration, 27*(9), 24–33.

6

LEADERSHIP AND DELEGATION

ELEMENTS OF LEADERSHIP AND DELEGATION

1. Defines and examines delegation

2. Discusses accountability

3. Offers real examples

4. Explores what makes a nurse leader

5. Considers the qualities you need in order to be a nurse leader

---

Though every RN is a leader, it may not come naturally to everyone. As a new registered nurse on the unit or in the organization, you may feel that you have no place in delegating to individuals who have more years of experience. It is vital to your success that you own your role as a leader and learn to delegate effectively. To help you succeed, this chapter will describe the ins and outs of delegation, as well as tips for building leadership skills.

Learning to Delegate

Delegation is an important part of being a registered nurse. For many reasons, you should delegate tasks to others: You will never be able to do everything for all of your patients all of the time. Delegating not only removes the burden of having to complete certain tasks but also lets the receiving person mature and experience new learning opportunities. You may have had an experience as a student when an RN was hesitant to allow you to perform certain tasks. This missed opportunity created a situation where your learning was hindered. Or you may have believed that the nurse lacked confidence in your ability to perform the tasks. You may never learn to do things if you are never given the opportunity.

What Is Delegation?

The American Nurses Association (ANA) and the National Council of State Boards of Nursing (NCSBN) joint statement considers *supervision* to be the delivery of guidance and the overseeing of a delegated nursing task (NCSBN.org, 2015). The registered nurse may complete the supervision by way of both written and verbal communication (NCSBN.org, 2015). The ANA's definition of *supervision* is the active process of directing, guiding, and influencing the outcomes of another person's performance of a specific task, whereas the NCSBN expresses *supervision* as the provision of leadership or direction, supervision, evaluation, and follow-up by the licensed nurse for the achievement of a delegated nursing task by an assistive employee (NCSBN.org, 2015). When you are supervising others, be sure that you understand the responsibility and accountability that you as the registered nurse assume.

The Ins and Outs of Delegation

Delegation requires the nurse's judgment and employs critical thinking and decision-making (Huber, 2014). The NCSBN (2015) states that delegation is a process that includes these four stages:

- Assess and plan.

- Communicate.

- Monitor and supervise.

- Evaluate and provide feedback.

When delegating a task, the nurse who is delegating and the person who is receiving the delegation must agree to the task, circumstances, timeframe, and feedback or progress for completion (Huber, 2014).

You may delegate to individuals with less education or more education than you have, depending on your role. As an RN in a team-based practice, you may be delegating to nursing assistants, LPNs/LVNs, other RNs, or unlicensed assistive personnel (UAPs). It is important that you understand their scope of practice if they are licensed so that you are not delegating a task or responsibility to them beyond their scope of practice.

Additionally, your team members need to be trained and competent to complete the task. To effectively delegate, you need to know the skills and abilities of those working with you. This may be difficult in an era where staff work 12-hour shifts and may not work with someone more than once a week or pay period. If you are ever uncomfortable about the skill or ability of a coworker, talk to your supervisor before you delegate a task or an assignment.

You may also be in a position sooner rather than later as the charge RN and be responsible for staffing assignments. Remember that you are delegating and that you need to understand the abilities, competencies, and skills of all team members working with you on that shift. Assigning the right staff to the right patients takes skill, but remember to always match the patient's needs with the RN's ability!

Remember that delegating is based on the patient's condition, the difficulty of the task, the expectedness of the outcomes, the abilities of the person to whom the task is delegated, and the context of the remaining patient needs (NCSBN, 2015).

THE PRINCIPLES OF DELEGATION

These are the five basic principles of delegation:

- The right task
- The right circumstances
- Delegate to the right person
- Provide the correct directions and communicate clearly
- Supervise and evaluate the outcome

(NCSBN.org, 2015)

Accountability and Responsibility

Nurses must also consider who holds the accountability and responsibility for the delegated task. Both the nurse who is delegating the task and the person who accepts the delegated task must verify that the proper information was communicated in an understandable manner and that the person assuming the delegation is competent to complete the task and hold the accountability. The responsibility lies with both individuals also: The nurse who is delegating must be responsible to evaluate whether the task was completed on time and correctly, and the person assuming the task is responsible for the notification and completion of the task on time and in the correct manner.

Often, RNs are afraid to delegate, feeling that their license is on the line if the individuals they delegate to do something wrong. If you delegate appropriately and individuals overshoot their scope or ability, fail to follow policies and procedures, or fail to report back to you appropriately, they will be the ones held accountable for errors or problems.

Delegation is learned over time and with practice. As a new nurse, you may not be proficient at delegating, but that should not keep you from delegating. Keep in mind that you may delegate tasks you personally could complete if you had the time, but delegating helps others mature professionally.

EXPERIENCE FROM THE FIELD: A SHORT HISTORY LESSON

As a new nurse, I was mainly interested in caring for patients. The sicker, the better, because the sicker the patient, the more I got to do. I had little to no interest in being in a leadership position. After all, the charge nurses had too many responsibilities in addition to carrying a patient load, and the nurse managers were always doing paperwork or attending a meeting. I wanted to be in on the action.

I started my nursing career as a licensed practical nurse (LPN). I had excellent skills training but absolutely no education in how to be a nurse leader. In the 1970s, it was not uncommon to be thrust into a leadership position by default; or, in other words, there was no one else to be the charge nurse for the shift. I was by nature a shy person, but a career in nursing had a way of bringing out the assertiveness I needed in order to assume a leadership role.

Over time, I realized that I was assuming more and more the charge nurse role on the evening or night shift and eventually became the charge nurse on the night shift in the emergency department of a small local hospital. I was responsible for everyone and everything on the unit. At that time, learning on the job was such common practice that most nurses never gave it a second thought, because rarely did nurses receive formal training in leadership and management.

Once I became a registered nurse, I realized my lack of knowledge and set out to do something about it. I found great mentors and coaches who truly made an impact on my career. I took on more responsibilities and went back to college to earn additional degrees that would better prepare me for a leadership role. I also became certified in my area of practice and nursing leadership and management.

–Cynthia M. Thomas, EdD, RN

Nurses as Leaders

Many nursing programs have now developed leadership/management courses to help prepare students for the transition to practice role. Healthcare organizations have also understood that great leaders must be properly educated and mentored, and we know of excellent organizations, such as the American Organization of Nurse Executives (AONE), which provides education and policies for nurse leaders; Sigma Theta Tau International (STTI), whose mission is to promote and develop leadership; and the American Nurses Association (ANA), which supports nurses at all levels of practice.

What Makes a Nurse Leader?

Huber (2014) explains that nursing is still a service profession whose mission is to care for and support people during both illness and wellness while serving as care providers and care coordinators. Nurse leaders may be formal or informal in style and tend to be visionaries, embracers of change, seekers of innovation, and leaders for patient-centered care. To be successful, leaders must also have the ability to delegate, to supervise others effectively, and to inspire confidence in others (Huber, 2014).

According to Guyton (2012), these nine principles can help to create outstanding nurse leaders:

Principle #1: Commit to excellence.

Principle #2: Measure the important things.

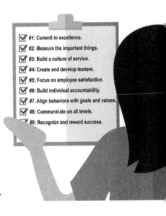

Principle #3: Build a culture of service.

Principle #4: Create and develop leaders.

Principle #5: Focus on employee satisfaction.

Principle #6: Build individual accountability.

Principle #7: Align behaviors with goals and values.

Principle #8: Communicate on all levels.

Principle #9: Recognize and reward success.

Though Guyton's principles were developed primarily for experienced nurse leaders, the same principles may be adapted and applied for new registered nurses. We have written our own version of Guyton's (2012) principles and adapted our principles for all nurses to develop and demonstrate noteworthy leadership skills regardless of the level of nursing practice.

Principle #1: Be Devoted to Excellence

Strive to be an excellent care provider, commit yourself to being a patient advocate, promote a culture of safety, endeavor to make a difference in others' lives, and remember to enjoy your passion for nursing. Embrace change, and always set an example for others to be a good role model. You never know when people are watching you and your behaviors.

Principle #2: Gauge the Significant Things

Identify what is truly important in your current job and in nursing as a profession. Be committed to your patients, your peers, the unit, the organization, and, most importantly, yourself. When you are at your best, everyone benefits.

Be honest with yourself and with your peers. Making a mistake may not be the end of your career; learn from the mistake and move forward. Be realistic about what you can accomplish, seek a mentor or coach, and openly share any concerns, frustrations, and accomplishments with others. Focus on safety and quality of care, always seek good role models to help you, and take care of yourself by having some "me time."

Principle #3: Create a Culture of Service

Guyton (2012) believes that nurses should appreciate patients and families as valuable customers. As customers, everyone wants to be acknowledged and served, especially when they are sick. Never ignore a patient or family member; always be ready to give a warm greeting. Better yet, make yourself the unit greeter. Anticipate the needs of patients, and always ask whether anything else is needed before exiting the room. Providing a time for your return may also reduce patient anxiety. If your unit is engaged in hourly or purposeful rounding, embrace it. Several studies indicate that hourly rounding increases patient satisfaction (Deitrick, Baker, Paxton, Flores, & Swavely, 2012; Halm, 2009).

POOR CULTURE OF SERVICE

To this day, I can clearly remember an incident that demonstrated a poor culture of service. I had just delivered my son and was being transferred to the mother/baby unit around 6:30 a.m. As the transporter and I were approaching the unit nursing station, I overheard a nurse say, "Oh, great—here comes another one. Why do they have to bring them close to shift change?" This incident occurred almost 40 years ago, but it is still fresh in my mind.

–Cindy Thomas, EdD, RN

Principle #4: Generate and Cultivate New Leaders

An experienced nurse once said, "There are leaders, and there are followers. There is a time to lead, and there is a time to follow." Think about this statement. We need great leaders. As older nurses retire, younger nurses will need to assume their leadership roles. Find a mentor or coach you are comfortable working with, and share your successes and frustrations. Over time, assume more and more responsibility to gain confidence as a nurse leader. Recognize that it is acceptable to delegate tasks to others. Delegating not only relieves you of tasks that others may take on but also helps others mature professionally.

We also need followers. We cannot have all leaders all the time. As a new nurse, you will need time to adjust to the unit and to your new role as a professional nurse. At times during this adjustment period, you may need to be a follower, rather than a leader, until you gain experience. Following applies to not only new nurses but also experienced nurses who may transfer to a new area of practice or who may be reentering practice.

Principle #5: Emphasize Employee Satisfaction

Excellent hospitals tend to have satisfied nurses (ANCC, 2014). It is up to everyone on staff to help create a satisfying work culture. Offer to help before someone asks. Truly get to know your peers. Be informed; recognize that it's acceptable to ask questions. If you are not happy with your work environment, consider transferring to another unit instead of leaving the organization or nursing profession. If you are unhappy with your current position and being transferred is unlikely, you may consider moving to a new organization. Sometimes, a move is necessary in order to continue learning and advancing in your career. Do everything you can to leave an organization on good terms, and never burn a bridge that you may have to cross again.

Principle #6: Be Accountable

Hold yourself and others accountable. If you offer to take a difficult assignment, don't complain later. Keep your commitment to work an additional shift. Arrive at work on time, prepared, and ready to do your best. Set an example to attend unit meetings and complete required continuing education early. If you witness others not following proper policies and procedures, talk to them about it. If confronting them makes you uncomfortable, discuss what you are seeing with the charge nurse or nurse manager. Remember that nurses do not work in isolation; it takes a team effort to provide safe, quality care to patients and a safe, rewarding environment in which to work.

Principle #7: Develop Great Goals and Values and Then Put Them into Action

Knowing the mission, vision, and values (philosophy) of the organization will help you to bring into line your behaviors to match. Explore your personal values: Your values may be challenged, and you will have to determine how to maintain them. Another aspect to consider is that your values may change over time, so periodic value checks are vital. Develop reasonable goals that can be achieved over time and that support the philosophy of the organization and help you to develop as a professional nurse. Always keep in mind that your values may or may not be shared by your patients and coworkers.

Principle #8: Communicate, Communicate, Communicate

Communication, one of the most important aspects of nursing, is integral to the nursing profession (Huber, 2014). Good communication prevents and reduces errors and promotes quality of care. Huber believes that proper communication is the key element for a nurse leader (2014). "Trust, respect, and empathy are the three ingredients needed to create and foster effective communication" (Huber, 2014, p. 111). Sullivan (2013) believes that effective communication is the key to success for nurse leaders. Communication differences also exist among generations of nurses; to avoid communication errors, you must recognize these differences (Sullivan, 2013).

Men and women also communicate differently, and because nurses work with interdisciplinary teams, you should recognize the differences in communication patterns, such as in these examples: Men believe that women ask too many questions; on the other hand, women do not feel included in men's conversations. Men like to receive personal recognition, and women prefer to be part of the team. Men retreat to solve issues, whereas women seek out others (Evans, 2014; Sullivan, 2013). Men tend to be more focused on the issue, and women relate more to personal experiences (Sullivan, 2013).

An excellent way to communicate important patient information is to use the SBAR-R method, or Situation, Background, Assessment, Recommendation, and Read back and Verify method (Thomas, Bertram, & Johnson, 2009). You can complete it in about 3 minutes. It has been proven quite effective.

SBAR-R

S = Situation—Quickly explain the problem, and keep it in mind while you communicate.

B = Background—Provide a brief background on the patient, and describe what has happened over the past 24 to 48 hours.

A = Assessment—Provide your current assessment of the patient.

R = Recommendation—Spell out your plan for the patient's care, including lab work, X-rays, and medication.

R = Read back and verify—Read back any information or orders that the physician provides to verify the information you have received and to avoid errors.

Principle #9: Acknowledge and Celebrate Achievement

Nurses often get so busy that they forget to recognize their successes. Rewards and recognition are important factors in helping to motivate and encourage nurses to continue their work, especially after difficult assignments. Good leaders are encouraging to others. Set the example by offering praises to your peers for a job well done. A simple thank you is so often appreciated by nurses because it shows that someone noticed and cared.

The nearby sidebar has a leadership checklist that you can follow.

LEADERSHIP CHECKLIST

- ❑ Be committed to others.
- ❑ Understand what is truly important.
- ❑ Serve others.
- ❑ Cultivate leadership.
- ❑ Work to develop both patient and self satisfaction.
- ❑ Be personally accountable.
- ❑ Develop realistic goals.
- ❑ Remain true to your values.
- ❑ Communicate well.
- ❑ Celebrate success.

The Essentials of Leadership Skills

Contrary to popular belief, it does take time to develop good leadership skills. Leaders are needed at all levels of nursing practice. Most acute and long-term care environments have team leaders, charge nurses, nurse managers, directors, and chief nursing officers. Poor leadership at any level can be detrimental to the quality of patient care and to patient and nurse satisfaction.

Leaders are essential. Leaders help to provide a balance in the needs of patients, the organization, nurses, physicians, and any other healthcare providers. To avoid burnout, leaders must also find an acceptable balance between work commitment and personal life (Sullivan, 2013).

You Can Be A Nurse Leader

Leadership is both formal and informal. Formal leaders have legitimate authority by way of their titles or job descriptions, whereas informal leaders may be assumed by careful and persuasive ideas that may influence the workflow (Sullivan, 2013). For example, a nurse who identifies a way to be more efficient while engaging in medication administration is demonstrating informal leadership.

What skills are needed to be an effective leader at any level of practice? Members of the American Organization of Nurse Executives (AONE, 2014) believe that managers at all levels of practice must be competent in the following areas. We have adapted the AONE competency levels for all nurses because we believe that all nurses may become great leaders at all levels of professional practice:

- Communication and the cultivation of relationships
- Knowledge of the healthcare setting
- Leadership skills
- Professionalism
- Business skills

Communication

The importance of good communication cannot be stressed enough. You must be able to communicate with other nurses and with physicians, patients, family members, and other care providers.

Nurses must communicate in both oral and written forms, in a timely fashion, with clarity, and at a high level of understanding while being concise.

You can and should build trusting relationships and collaboration with nurses, physicians, and other healthcare disciplines by employing these simple techniques:

- Communicate to the right people at the right time and in the right manner.

- Follow through on your promises.

- Do everything in your power to give excellent care and to be a positive member of the team.

- Develop empathy and sympathy and compassion for others, but also develop self-compassion because you must take care of yourself before you can care for others (Neff, 2015).

- Be assertive but in a nonthreatening and nonjudgmental manner.

- Embrace diversity, learn about different cultures, and share what you learn with others.

- Share in the decision-making process by serving on unit and organizational committees, sharing your opinions, and welcoming the opinions of others.

- Participate in or create community outreach and service programs.

- Communicate positively about the nursing profession, and take ownership of the nursing profession, because it starts with each nurse.

Knowing Your Healthcare Environment

Being knowledgeable of the healthcare environment means more than showing up for work and doing your job. You must also:

- Know and understand the nurse practice act in your state.

- Apply best patient care standards to your practice.

- Commit yourself to evidence-based practice, and participate in studies whenever possible.

- Make yourself familiar with the organizational policy and procedures.

- Ensure safety by employing safety practices for your patient, yourself, and your team members.

- Understand and utilize the case management system.

- Participate in the organization's quality management programs.

- Minimize the risks and liabilities to you and the organization by adhering to the organization's quality and safety protocols.

Developing Leadership Skills

To be an effective leader, you must develop good leadership skills:

- Explore how you make decisions and determine what elements affect the decisions you make.

- Examine your personal belief systems and how they might affect your decision-making ability.

- Be willing to explore new ways of doing things.

- Think big; let your outlook surpass the here and now, and broaden your views and practice to a more global level.

- Be reflective and willing to make changes.

- Commit to lifelong learning.

- Seek out helpful mentors.

- Value feedback to improve your practice.

- Be loyal and committed to your organization.

- Promote the profession of nursing.

- Serve as a role model to others.

- Embrace change and adapt to the situation at hand.

Being Professional

You must also consider these areas of professionalism if you want to be an effective leader:

- Hold yourself and others accountable for actions.

- Set reasonable expectations, goals, and objectives.

- Start now to develop a progressive career path; it might include continuing education for a graduate degree or certification in your area of practice.

- As you gain experience, serve as a mentor, preceptor, or coach.

- Always maintain a professional behavior and appearance, and remember that first impressions do count.

- Maintain the highest ethics every single day; your conduct should follow your high standards. Develop good credibility.

- Promote evidence-based practices.

- Be an advocate for not only your patients but also the nursing profession.

- Join and be an active member of a favorite nursing professional organization.

- Do not engage in violent behaviors such as bullying, ignoring others, or refusing to help.

Honing Good Business Skills

To be a leader, you must develop good business skills. You may wonder why you need these skills if you are not the manager, but all nurses should be business-savvy. Healthcare is a business, and everyone must participate to make the business successful.

These strategies can help you develop your business skills:

- Read the organizational chart to know how your organization functions.

- Avoid being wasteful with supplies and your time.

- Be a recruiter for your organization; tell others about the positive environment and encourage them to become employees.

- Never engage in practices that would result in negative publicity for the organization: Don't post on social media sites or gossip about an employee or the organization or violent behaviors, for example.

- Understand the role of technology in healthcare and use it to your advantage.

Remember that all RNs are leaders. Embrace your role as a leader, and learn more about leadership skills. They will become useful in all avenues of your life, personally and professionally.

Chapter Checkup

Key points from this chapter include:

- ❏ Delegation and supervision are important aspects of being a registered nurse.

- ❏ To delegate effectively, you need to know the skills and abilities of those working with you.

- ❏ Memorize the five basic principles of delegation.

- ❏ All RNs are leaders, regardless of position.

- ❏ Leadership is both formal and informal.

- ❏ Be professional at all times.

- ❏ Know your organization.

- ❏ Strive toward leadership.

- ❏ Develop good business sense.

References

American Nurses Credentialing Center (ANCC). (2014). Frequently asked questions about ANCC's Magnet Recognition Program. Retrieved from http://www.nursecredentialing.org/Magnet/International/MagnetProgOverview/MagnetProgFAQ.html

American Organization of Nurse Executives (AONE). (2014). The AONE nurse executive competencies. Retrieved from http://www.aone.org/resources/leadership%20tools/nursecomp.shtml

Deitrick, L. M., Baker, K., Paxton, H., Flores, M., & Swavely, D. (2012). Hourly rounding: Challenges with implementation of an evidence-based process. *Journal of Nursing Care Quality*, 27(1), 13–19.

Evans, L. (2014). Are we speaking a different language? Men and women's communication blind spots. Retrieved from http://www.fastcompany.com/3031631/strong-female-lead/are-we-speaking-a-different-language-men-and-womens-communication-blind-s

Guyton, N. (2012). Nine principles of successful nursing leadership. *American Nurse Today, 7*(8). Retrieved from www.americannursetoday.com/nine-principles-of-successful-nursing-leadership

Halm, M. A. (2009). Hourly rounds: What does the evidence indicate? *American Journal of Critical Care, 18*(6), 581–584. doi:20.4037/ajcc2009350

Huber, D. L. (2014). *Leadership & nursing care management* (5th ed.). St. Louis, MO: Elsevier Saunders.

NCSBN.org. (2015). National Council of State Boards of Nursing joint statement on delegation. American Nurses Association and NCSBN. Retrieved from https://www.ncsbn.org/Delegation_joint_statement_NCSBN-ANA.pdf

Neff, K. (2015). Self-compassion. Retrieved from http://self-compassion.org/the-three-elements-of-self-compassion-2/

Sullivan, E. J. (2013). *Effective leadership and management in nursing* (8th ed.). Upper Saddle River, NJ: Pearson Education.

Thomas, C. M., Bertram, E., & Johnson, D. (2009). The SBAR communication technique. *Nurse Educator, 34*(4), 176–180. doi:10.1097/NNE.0b013e3181aaba54. PMID 19574858

7

RELIEVING STRESS

ELEMENTS OF RELIEVING STRESS

1. Charts the impact of stress

2. Examines the reasons for stress

3. Describes different types of stress

4. Explains compassion fatigue

5. Provides strategies for work life effectiveness

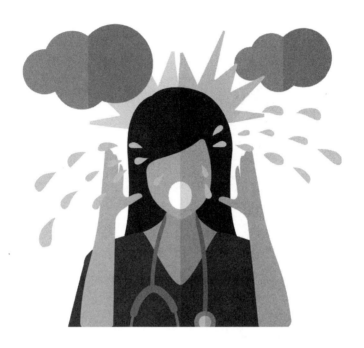

Most people experience some stress, which can be beneficial and even essential to life (Sullivan, 2013). You might even be experiencing some stress right now. Stress can help your performance, but stress can also hinder your performance (Sullivan, 2013). It is very important to understand the different types of stressors and how to reduce specific stressors in your life. Rosenthal (2002) defines *stress* as a negative emotional experience linked with biological changes that prompt the body to adapt. Severe and chronic stress can produce health problems and may lead to burnout (Huber, 2014). You may have thought that after graduating from college, you would see all your stress disappear. The reality is that it will always be part of your life. You can use stress to your benefit by learning to balance stress.

Examining the Reasons Behind Stress

Registered nurses (RNs) face job-related stress (organizational) and personal stress (intrapersonal and interpersonal), and they all affect their ability to function at their best (Sullivan, 2013).

Organizational Stress

Organizational stress, which is job-related, may come from a variety of sources such as role ambiguity (not having a clearly defined role or expectation) and role conflict (how you determine your role and how the role is really determined). Role conflict may also result from being employed as a student tech before assuming the role of the RN on the same unit. Many new RNs struggle at first to step out of the student tech role and into the professional nurse role, and many nurse peers fail to recognize the change in roles from student to professional nurse, which creates role conflict (Sullivan, 2013).

A person with organizational stress may experience feeling over-loaded by an assignment, unprepared to take on a more difficult assignment, or unable to find clear or sufficient information. The physical environment can also produce stress when the lighting is poor, when supplies for a job are missing, or when you have feelings of being unsafe—or you experience constant noise, a lack of space, a disorganized environment, or little time for meals or breaks, for example (Sullivan, 2013).

Interpersonal Stress

Nurses, who rarely work alone, are most often working in collaboration with many other healthcare professionals. This collaboration may also produce stress because everyone has a specific role within the realm of providing care to the patient. Nurses are also being burdened with additional tasks as organizations seek to find new ways to lower costs and reduce the number of employees. Not everyone works the same or has the same values or work ethics, which may create conflict among employees and eventually lead to stress.

Intrapersonal Stress

Most people like to think that they can leave their personal problems at home while they go to work, but in reality it is generally not possible. The best strategy is to recognize your personal stressors and respond to them appropriately. Everyday stressors are at work whether you are experiencing marital status or major relationship changes, additions to your family unit, home relocation, additional family caregiving responsibilities, major illness amongst loved ones, and financial challenges. As a new RN, you might experience *reality shock*, a syndrome often experienced when a student is transitioning to the professional nurse role (Kramer, 1974).

People who feel overloaded with stress or unable to handle stress may develop prolonged anxiety, phobias, and persistent states of fear, often hindering their ability to work or function daily. Many individuals suffer from depression and may withdraw from associating with peers and family. They may have mood or behavior changes as well as physical symptoms such as hypertension, headaches, ulcers, arthritis, heart disease, or eating disorders. Additionally, some people may turn to illegal drugs, prescription medications, or alcohol (Epstein, 2010; Sullivan, 2013). An overall result of the inability to deal with constant stress is burnout, resulting in feelings of being unable to do the job (Epstein, 2010).

Compassion Fatigue

Compassion fatigue is a more recent phenomenon that is experienced by caregivers and is similar to post-traumatic stress disorder (Newsom, 2010; Yoder, 2010). Nurses may experience symptoms like burnout, but the symptoms may be on a more severe level, especially if the nurse is working in high-stress areas such as emergency departments or intensive care units (Gates, Gillespie, & Succop, 2011). As a result of developing compassion fatigue, many nurses may feel inadequate and leave their jobs or the nursing profession. Joinson (1992) described compassion fatigue as being unique to people in the caregiver role.

Similar to experiencing burnout, nurses might experience dread in caring for specific patients or have decreased empathy or increased use of sick time, decreased joy, physical illnesses, or emotional issues (Lombardo & Eyre, 2011). Identifying the resources available in the work environment is an important step to recovery. Many organizations offer an employee assistance program (EAP) or pastoral care for a variety of issues employees might be experiencing. Counselors may provide support and help develop strategies to overcome compassion fatigue. Lombardo and Eyre (2011) also suggest that nurses seek a mentor or a peer in the workplace who may be more understanding and familiar with the work situation to help identify realistic strategies and promote a better work-life balance.

EXPERIENCE FROM THE FIELD: SO MUCH BLEEDING

I was shaking as I left the hospital to drive home. All I could think about was the blood—my patient was losing a large amount of blood after the birth of her first baby. Her husband sat unaware, totally absorbed in rocking their newborn nearby. It was my fifth day on orientation as a new nurse on a labor-and-delivery unit, and I had just witnessed a postpartum hemorrhage (PPH) for the first time.

Despite having had a long and complicated labor and delivery, the new mother was recovering normally after delivering her baby. Unfortunately, after about an hour the young patient's condition changed. She started vomiting, her vital signs changed, and her vaginal bleeding increased. My preceptor and I notified the patient's doctor, who quickly responded to evaluate the patient.

From that moment on, everything was a blur. It all seemed to be happening so quickly yet in slow motion. While the doctor was examining the patient, she began bleeding even more. As I watched, I felt a sense of panic in my chest. My heart was racing. I remember asking the patient's husband to move from his chair at the foot of the bed to the couch nearby because I didn't want him to see what was happening.

I knew my patient was in trouble, but I didn't know exactly how to help. I was brand-new to the unit, and this was my first time to experience a true emergency. I didn't yet know where supplies were located or which step to take next. The only thing I could do was stand at the head of my patient's bed, hold her hand, and try to keep her calm. While I was doing this, my preceptor showed that she knew exactly what to do: She calmly yet swiftly intervened, calling for extra help and retrieving medications to help stop the patient's bleeding.

After a few minutes, the doctor determined that the patient needed to return to the operating room because she was losing too much blood. My preceptor notified the charge nurse and started quickly preparing the patient for a transfer. The room was instantly filled with staff. As the physician and anesthesiologist spoke to the patient and her family, I heard terms such as possible hysterectomy, blood transfusion, and lifesaving measures. As we rushed out of the room, I caught the eye of the patient's mother, whom I had chatted with throughout the day. She said to me: "Take care of my baby."

We raced to the operating room (OR), where a team waited. It was my first time in an OR. I was struck by how bright and cold the room seemed. Everyone moved quickly and efficiently, and everyone had a job to do—except me. I stood alone, nearly in shock. Thankfully, the mask I wore hid my fearful expression. I remained with my patient and kept her attention focused on me. I calmly reassured her that we would take good care of her and that I would hold her hand until she was asleep.

While everyone finished their preparation around me, I stayed with the patient until she was safely under anesthesia. Then I stood back and watched the team work. The doctor was able to quickly identify the cause of the bleeding and stop it. Shift change occurred toward the end of the procedure, and my team handed over our patient to the next crew of capable nurses.

I was not present to see my patient awaken in the recovery room, but I left my shift knowing that she was leaving that OR with her uterus. I knew that the child she had just given birth to would not be the only one she could ever carry and that her husband, her new baby, and her family would not have to leave the hospital without her. She would not be one of the women who die every day in the United States from complications of childbirth.

I left the hospital, shaken up after my shift. I was not afraid of what I had seen—I was afraid that I didn't know how to respond to it. I realized that I was having a normal reaction to an abnormal circumstance, but I didn't like feeling powerless to recover. I knew that I never wanted to repeat this feeling, and I promised myself that the next time it happened, I would be ready.

From that night on, I learned as much as I could about PPH. I sought out evidence-based research, attended outside webinars, familiarized myself with risk factors, learned the early signs of PPH, studied unit policies and procedures, practiced quickly removing PPH medications from the med cart, memorized the location of the emergency carts, and read literature produced by my professional nursing organization. I still have a lot to learn, but I know much more now than I did on that fifth day of orientation.

The next day, as my preceptor and I went to visit the patient, tears filled my eyes the moment I walked into her room. She looked wonderful! She was sitting up in bed and eating dinner while her baby napped nearby in the bassinet. Her husband and mother raced across the room to hug us. Her mother wrapped her arms around me and said, between sobs, "Thank you for taking care of my baby!" I was ecstatic to be able to say, "I told you we would."

My belief as a new nurse was reinforced: Even though I had graduated from nursing school and successfully passed the NCLEX, I've only scratched the surface of what I need to know to become an expert nurse. I know that knowledge and comfort will increase as I practice, but I owe it to my patients, their families, and myself to seek out information beyond what I learned in school.

It is a privilege to be a labor-and-delivery nurse. Helping birth a baby, watching a woman become a mother, handing a father his child to hold for the first time, and seeing an older sibling fawn over a new baby brother or sister are some of the great honors of my life. It is my job to do my best to ensure that a baby doesn't leave the hospital without its mother or that a new father doesn't have to raise his child alone without the mom who lovingly carried their child. The time for learning does not end with graduation; it has only just started.

I have also learned that the quiet and confident new nurse is the one who most worries the experienced nurses. A new nurse should be curious, willing to ask for help, open to constructive criticism, and receptive of every opportunity to learn from more senior nurses. Though evidence-based research is the gold standard for acquiring knowledge, much can be learned from peers in the same way they learned from the nurses who preceded them.

After this incident, I debriefed with my preceptor so that I could better understand what had transpired. I continually ask experienced nurses questions, and I try to attend every birth I can so that I can watch other nurses in action. This event, though terrifying, was a defining moment in my young career, and it inspired me to always seek new knowledge. As Maya Angelou said: "I did then what I knew how to do. Now that I know better, I do better."

—JA, BSN, RN

Work-Life Effectiveness

Becoming a new nurse is truly exciting. Along with that excitement comes a bit of apprehension and, honestly, perhaps some fear. Feeling uncertain is a normal part of entering the professional nursing practice and acclimating to the RN role. Some nurses (maybe even you) find it difficult to balance their work and home lives, because they work too many hours. They may need the extra money to pay off student loans, buy a new car, or even upgrade their living spaces. New nurses may simply enjoy making money so they tend to work more than others. You may find it difficult to say no when asked to work overtime or feel that you have an obligation to work extra hours. To be a successful, healthy nurse, you must create a balance of work and personal time. You may need to simply say, "No."

EXPERIENCE FROM THE FIELD: WHEN TO SAY NO

I remember the excitement of my first few weeks as an official registered nurse, working on a medical-surgical unit. Fresh from the NCLEX, I wanted to help people, connect with my patients, and aid in the healing process. That's what draws people to the nursing profession, right? People pursue it because they are innate caregivers. It isn't the part that is taught in nursing school; it is the part that dwells in every fiber of a nurse's being. It's what makes us the most trusted profession in the Gallup polls.

The patients know that nurses are putting them first, but who is taking care of nurses? If you've ever taken an airline flight, you've no doubt heard the routine speech of the flight attendants: "Place the oxygen mask on your own face before assisting those around you." This strategy seems so logical, yet nurses regularly fail to embrace it. They travel from one patient room to the next, holding their collective breath as they care for the needs of, and relieve the pains of, others while ignoring those of their own bodies. That is who nurses are, but not who they must be. Eleanor Brownn said, "Rest and self-care are so important. When you take time to replenish your spirit, it allows you to serve others from the overflow. You cannot serve from an empty vessel."

If I could impart only a single piece of advice to the new nurse, it is to remember to care for yourself. Compassion fatigue is at the root of many instances of nurse burnout, and in some cases, of substance abuse issues. In my own career, I reached the point where I considered leaving the nursing profession. Though I could have never identified the problem of compassion fatigue at the time, I knew that I was exhausted and lacking the joy I had earlier felt in my work.

The problem was that I had forgotten to put on my mask first. Now I care for myself daily with meditation and mindfulness-based practices, freeing myself to be in the moment with my patients throughout my shift and to leave the concerns of the day at my place of work when I go home.

My vessel is now full. I am reenergized by my daily self-care practice and am again passionate about my work as an RN. What fills your heart and restores your soul may be different from my meditation practice. Some nurses I know find their energy in roller derby or artwork. The type of care you provide for yourself is less important than the fact that you simply provide it. Caring for yourself must be intentional. You must place that oxygen mask and breathe deeply. Take the time to give yourself the same love and attention as you bestow on your patients. It is, after all, who you are.

–Jenna Sanders, MSN, RN

This chapter highlights the types of stress nurses may encounter daily regardless of how experienced the nurse is. Follow these strategies to avoid unnecessary stress and help lower stress when it arises.

These strategies can help you avoid creating unnecessary stress:

- **Prioritize**—Organize your to-do list to avoid running late and increasing your stress level.

- **Delegate**—Do not attempt to do everything yourself. Hand off burdensome tasks and assignments to increase productivity and improve communication while building teams.

- **Communicate while compromising**—A fellow healthcare professional (for example, RN, MD, CEO) might want your attention at the exact moment you are completing a nursing intervention. Simply communicating could avoid stress. "I would be happy to give you all my attention after I finish this treatment to my patient."

- **Know your resources**—No nurse works alone. Many types of resources are available, including policy/procedure manuals, peers, and supervisors who can assist in finding information.

- **Just say no**—See the earlier sidebar titled "Experience From the Field: When to Say No."

These strategies can help you lower stress:

- **Change the scenery**—If allowed by your employer's policies, take food breaks off the floor.

- **Take 10 and breathe**—Counting to 10 while breathing deeply can reduce stress by lowering your heart rate and blood pressure. It can also put you in a better frame of mind to deal with a stressful situation.

- **Develop a healthy lifestyle**—Follow a proper diet, get lots of exercise, and drink plenty of water.

- **Get plenty of rest before reporting to work.**

- **Communicate with fellow employees**—Stress can also be caused by harboring frustrations or bad feelings. Don't let a problem fester. Deal with it and move on.

Chapter Checkup

Key points from this chapter include:

- ❑ You will always experience some stress as a nurse.

- ❑ Some stress is good for you.

- ❑ There are three main types of stress: organizational, interpersonal, and intrapersonal.

- ❑ To reduce stress, you must understand what causes stress for you.

- ❑ Compassion fatigue is unique to healthcare providers, especially nurses, and is similar to post-traumatic stress disorder.

- ❑ Find a balance between work and personal time.

- ❑ Follow proven stress-reducing strategies.

References

Epstein, D. G. (2010). Extinguish workplace stress. *Nursing Management, 41*(10), 34–37.

Gates, D. M., Gillespie, G. L., & Succop, P. (2011). Violence against nurses and its impact on stress and productivity. *Nursing Economics, 29*(2), 59–66.

Huber, D. L. (2014). *Leadership and nursing care management* (5th ed.). St. Louis, MO: Elsevier-Saunders.

Joinson, C. (1992). Coping with compassion fatigue. *Nursing, 22*(4), 116, 118–119, 120.

Kramer, M. (1974). *Reality shock*. St. Louis, MO: Mosby.

Lombardo, B., & Eyre, C. (2011). Compassion fatigue: A nurse's primer. *The Online Journal of Issues in Nursing, 16*(1). doi: 10.3912/OJIN.Vol16No01Man03

Newsom, R. (2010). Compassion fatigue: Nothing left to give. *Nursing Management, 41*(4), 42–45.

Rosenthal, M. S. (2002). *50 ways to prevent and manage stress*. New York, NY: McGraw-Hill.

Sullivan, E. J. (2013). *Effective leadership and management in nursing*. Boston, MA: Pearson.

Yoder, E. A. (2010). Compassion fatigue in nurses. *Applied Nursing Research, 23*(4), 191–197.

BEING SAFE: DEALING WITH INJURIES/VIOLENCE IN THE WORKPLACE

ELEMENTS OF BEING SAFE:
DEALING WITH INJURIES/VIOLENCE
IN THE WORKPLACE

1. Examines the types of violence nurses face

2. Considers the causes of that violence

3. Covers strategies to reduce violence

4. Identifies victim violence

5. Provides case studies for reflections

As you transition to the registered nurse (RN) role or to a new role within the professional practice, you may encounter some difficult people who exhibit a variety of violent behaviors. Healthcare is not immune to violence. As a nurse you are interacting with many people who are ill, under stress, anxious, under the influence of drugs or alcohol, living with mental health disorders, or fearful of the future. Patients, family members, and even your peers may not handle stress well or may become overwhelmed by the pressures of difficult situations. You may have already experienced or witnessed violent behaviors from a patient, family member, or, sadly, another nurse or physician. Our goal in this chapter is to alert you to the many forms of violence in healthcare and provide strategies to reduce or defuse the behaviors.

Types of Workplace Violence

Violence in the workplace is not new, and nursing is not an exception to violence. In fact, workplace violence occurs in healthcare more often than it does in any other workplace environment (Howard & Gilboy, 2009). In 2013, Speroni, Fith, Dawson, Dugan, and Atherton found that 76% of nurses reported experiencing a verbal or physical attack (2013). The United States Bureau of Labor Statistics (2010) reported healthcare employees were the victims of over 11,370 assaults, a 13% increase since 2009. Violence in the workplace is considered to be acts of physical and verbal assaults and threats aimed toward a person while that person is at work (Howard & Gilboy, 2009). There were at least 2,130 assaults occurring in nursing and residential care facilities, and assaults are most likely a higher number since many assaults are not reported.

The assaults can inflict physical or emotional harm to employees, visitors, and patients (McPhaul & Lipscomb, 2008; Papa & Venella, 2013). Though much of the violence comes from patients, nurse-to-nurse violence is one of the highest forms, followed by physician-to-nurse (Thomas, 2010).

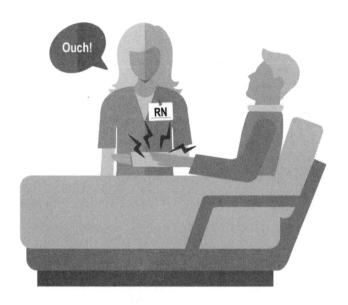

Violence comes in many fashions (see Table 8.1), including threatening behaviors, verbal and written statements, and physical attacks of biting, hitting, kicking, shoving, throwing things, and pushing people (Sullivan, 2013). More violent behaviors might include the use of guns or knives, rape, sexual harassment, or murder (Sullivan, 2013).

There are many names for violence in the workplace, such as *lateral violence, horizontal violence,* and *bullying* (Thomas, 2010). Many states are taking a more proactive approach to stopping violence in healthcare facilities by making it a felony to assault or commit battery against emergency department nurses (Trotto, 2014). There is a drive to have Congress pass legislation for increased preparation for, recognition of, and de-escalating of violent behaviors in healthcare organizations (Trotto, 2014).

Table 8.1   Common Types of Workplace Violence

Nurse-to-Nurse	Physician-to-Nurse	Patient-to-Nurse
Yelling in the nursing station, hallway, or patient room	Throwing things at a person or in a room	Kick, a physical act
Not acknowledging a request by simply avoiding or walking away from the person	Making derogatory remarks toward a person or to others	Hit, a physical act
Sighing, a covert action (not openly displaying behavior)	Making sexual comments to a person or to others	Biting, a physical act
Eye rolling, a covert action (not openly displaying behavior)	Yelling directly or indirectly to the person	Throwing things, a physical act
Gossiping about the person to others	Hanging up on a phone call	Threatening a person directly or indirectly
Making rude comments to a person or to others	Making demeaning remarks directly or indirectly to the person	Using guns, knives, or other weapons directly or indirectly on the person
Threatening someone	Making a person the brunt of jokes directly or indirectly	Calling the person names or referring negatively to gender, sexual orientation, or ethicality
Excluding someone from the team	Making threatening comments directly to the person	

What Causes Violence?

The nurse's job can at times be stressful. Nurses often work 12-hour shifts in difficult situations. They are working with a variety of people with different personalities and coping mechanisms, and often people have unrealistic expectations of nurses and other healthcare providers. When people are sick, they frequently behave differently. Patients and family members may exhibit a fear of the unknown and lash out in frustration.

Gates, Gillespie, and Succop (2011) believe that working in healthcare increases the risks for violent behaviors, much of it being created by stress. In addition, emergency departments are prone to violent behaviors by nature of psychiatric and confused patients, alcohol and drug abusers, and violent patients such as murderers and gang members (Gates et al., 2011; Wood & Brott, 2013). Psychiatric departments and hospitals, emergency departments, geriatric facilities such as Alzheimer's facilities, and overcrowded waiting rooms are potential areas for increased violent events (Nachreiner et al., 2007). Additionally, nurses who work alone or with limited staff, who work in areas with longer waiting times, and who spend time in less secure spaces like parking lots and dimly lit areas are at increased risk of violent behaviors (Glacki-Smith et al., 2010; Sullivan, 2013).

Reducing the Risk of Being a Victim of Violence

No one should be subjected to violent behaviors regardless of the magnitude of the behavior. The workplace should be a safe environment that is free from intimidation and fear. Nurses should not hesitate to ask questions and seek help when needed.

The Joint Commission mandated that all healthcare organizations have a zero-tolerance policy and procedure in place to address and eliminate violence from the work environment (The Joint Commission, 2012). You can review this

 Realistically, policies are effective only if the people working within the organization are willing to enforce them. Be willing to report someone who is bullying or displaying violent behaviors toward you.

policy at http://www.jcrinc.com/assets/1/7/ECNews-Jan-2012.pdf. Knowing your organization's policies and procedures on violence is vital and helps to protect you as a potential victim.

Nurses must know the warning signs of an impending violent event and be able to either defuse it or get help. Consider these great tips to recognize violent warning signs when someone:

- Stands close or moves aggressively toward you

- Yells or escalates his or her voice when you attempt to talk to the person

- Elevates his or her arms in a fighting or striking position

- Stares blankly or appears disconnected

- Clenches or hits his or her fists

- Possesses or brandishes a weapon of any type: pen, knife, gun, heavy object, or even a patient chart

- Makes angry comments such as "I'm going to kill you" or "I'm going to knock your brains out" or "I'll be waiting for you in the parking lot"

- Attempts to prevent you from leaving or moving out of the way by standing in front of you or barring the door or exit

- Bars you from retreating to a safe place (Sullivan, 2013; Wood & Brott, 2013)

Following are the steps you can take in these situations to protect yourself and others:

- Do not approach or try to take a weapon from a person.

- Do not turn your back on the person, but slowly walk backward, keeping your vision on the person at all times.

- Call Security or 911, or call out for help or for someone else to call 911 or Security.

- Remain calm and avoid threatening a violent person, slow your breathing, and change the subject, if necessary.

- Protect other patients, close other patient room doors, lock unit or office doors, and direct people away from the area.

- Do not allow the violent person to be close to the door if in a room; remain by the door so that you can exit quickly if needed.

- Move to a safe area. (Sullivan, 2013; Wood & Brott, 2013)

Report abusers immediately, using the appropriate steps in your organization.

The Not-So-Obvious Workplace Violence

The sad fact is that violence is a negative part of healthcare, and nurses must learn how to recognize and protect themselves from falling victim to such behaviors. Most nurses have been subjected to some form of violence during their careers (Speroni et al., 2013; Thomas, 2010). Maybe you have also, but brushed it off as just part of the job. The incident may be as simple as another nurse rolling her eyes when asked a question or reach the level of bearing witness to a physician throwing a chart or personally experiencing sexual harassment.

New nurses are especially vulnerable to violence but may not recognize it as such (Thomas, 2010). Some not-so-obvious violent behaviors are someone giving the silent treatment, sighing, walking away when approached, refusing to help when asked, giving angry looks, and excluding others. Consider the following examples of not-so-obvious bullying incidents.

The Eye Roll

What it is: You may recall as a child rolling your eyes whenever your parents told you to do something you didn't want to do. It was a subtle covert action that indicated your displeasure with something.

Example: Mary, a new nurse, asks Bill, an experienced nurse, for help to program an IV infusion machine. Bill rolls his eyes so that other nurses can see his objection to the request and pretends that he does not hear Mary.

Ways to deal with it: Mary should confront Bill about the incident. Mary is confronting Bill's behavior, not Bill personally. Mary might say something like this: "I know I ask for help often, but I am still learning. You are the best nurse to help me because you are so good with problems like troubleshooting the IV machines." This statement lets Bill know that Mary values his help and expertise and potentially defuses a violent behavior.

Ignoring

What it is: Ignoring happens when you make a request or ask a question to another person who does not acknowledge you or the request.

Example: Rose, an LPN, was floated to the 4South medical unit today. She has never worked on this unit and is unsure of the routines. Rose asks Connie, one of the regular unit nurses, when vital signs are generally taken. Connie responds by simply ignoring Rose. In fact, Connie gets up and walks out of the nursing station without addressing Rose's question.

Ways to deal with it: One way to deal with ignoring situations is to confront the person about the behavior. You might say something like this: "I have never worked on this unit, and I am willing to do whatever work I am qualified to do, but I need some initial direction about the unit routine. Would you be willing to answer some of my questions?"

The Angry Doctor/Teammate

What it is: Dr. Jackson is well known for his difficult behaviors, and in fact, many nurses simply accept his behaviors and pass along this advice: "Well, that's just how he is, and you will get used to him."

Example: Sally, an RN, is assisting Dr. Jackson with a bedside lumbar puncture procedure. Dr. Jackson asks for a medication that is not normally given during the procedure and is not among the medications in the room. Sally informs him that she will have to leave the room or call another nurse to obtain the medication, which will delay the procedure. Dr. Jackson lashes out at Sally, yelling and cursing that she should have been more prepared and he will report her to the nurse manager.

Ways to deal with it: Sally should not accept the abusive behavior that Dr. Jackson is displaying. An appropriate response would be for Sally to calmly state, "Dr. Jackson, I will not accept being cursed at or yelled at by you. If I had been notified prior to the procedure that you might want that particular medication, I would have ensured it was present. If I step out of the room to obtain the medication, it might present a safety issue for the patient; therefore, I will call another nurse to obtain the medication as soon as possible."

Excluded from the Team

What it is: Being excluded from the team is another form of violence. It implies that you are not worthy, that you are not part of us, that we don't care about you. Being excluded may result in a hostile work environment.

Example: Cheryll was a new registered nurse working the night shift on a busy medical surgical unit. The more experienced nurses had all been working together on the unit for at least 6 years and were friends outside the organization as well. Cheryll had never felt part of the team, because the nurses tended to exclude her from conversations or not invite her to social events outside of work.

Ways to deal with it: The unit was particularly busy one night with several new admissions from the emergency department. Cheryll had completed only two admission assessments on her own and was concerned about her ability to complete the admission assessment on a patient with multiple acute health issues and family members with lots of questions. She decided to seek help from Beth, one of the more experienced nurses, who was sitting at the nursing station.

When Cheryll asked Beth for help completing the admission assessment, Beth pretended she did not hear Cheryll and walked out of the nursing station. Frustrated, Cheryll decided to find Beth and ask her again for help. As she approached a patient room, Cheryll overheard Beth talking about her to another nurse on the unit. "She is so stupid. What did they teach this girl in nursing school, anyway? She can't do anything for herself. I wish they would have never hired her. She doesn't fit in."

Subsequently, Cheryll went back to her patient room and completed the admission assessment on her own. The next evening when she reported to work, the nurse manager asked to meet with her. Cheryll was given a written warning, composed by Beth, for making an error of omission for a routine medication the patient had been taking before the hospital stay. Cheryll was so upset that she resigned her position to evaluate whether she should remain a nurse.

Being excluded from the team can be very difficult. Exclusion is also a form of violence because it sets the person apart and sends the message "You are not one of us." Cheryll should have confronted the nurse's actions and explained that she is new to nursing and to the unit and needs help from experienced nurses. If Cheryll believes the nurse's actions are creating a hostile work environment, she would need to make a formal complaint to the nurse manager. Though it is not required that a nurse is included in personal activities outside of the work environment and it is not necessary that everyone likes everyone else, nurses must be respectful to each other and work as a team or a cohesive group to maintain a safe, quality work environment.

Workplace Injuries

Many injuries are the result of workplace violence and need to be addressed to bring awareness and to support education and prevention programs. Other situations happen in healthcare organizations resulting in workplace injuries that may have been prevented. Nevertheless, nurses must be aware of potential risk factors in healthcare organizations to minimize their risk of injury.

Knowing how to avoid injuries and employ proper safety techniques for yourself and your patients is vital. Not surprisingly, injuries such as in the back and neck occur most often in healthcare environments and are estimated to cost more than $7 billion every year (Nordqvist, 2013). The American Nurses Association (ANA) statement makes it clear that back, neck, and shoulder injuries are preventable with the proper education and equipment (Nordqvist, 2013).

Many types of injuries can happen in healthcare organizations. The Centers for Disease Control and Prevention (CDC) reported that healthcare workplace injuries included needle sticks, latex allergies, back and neck injuries, violence, stress, exposure to chemicals, disease, and illnesses such as blood-borne pathogens (2014a). Nonfatal injuries in healthcare rank among the highest of any industry (CDC, 2014a).

The law mandates, though it may be difficult, that employers provide a safe environment for workers. The nature of healthcare predisposes nurses to viruses, bacteria, and a large number of illnesses. Exposure to needle stick injuries places nurses at risk for the hepatitis B and C viruses as well as for human immunodeficiency virus (HIV) (CDC, 2014b).

We tend to think of sharps primarily as needles, yet nurses work in a variety of places and are exposed to a multitude of sharp items. Among the more common are scalpels, lancets, razor blades, scissors, wire, retractors, clamps, pins, staples, cutters, and glass (Canadian Centre for Occupational Health and Safety [CCOHS], 2014). Some diseases contracted through sharps injuries are brucellosis, diphtheria, cutaneous gonorrhea, herpes, malaria, staphylococcus, syphilis, toxoplasmosis, and tuberculosis (CCOHS, 2014).

Unfortunately, sharps are often easily accessible to someone intent on harming another person. It would not be particularly difficult to pull used syringes from a needle box hanging on a wall, use the foam antiseptic spray to temporarily blind someone, or grab some lancets to stab another person. Heavy or falling equipment, burns, and inhalants can also injure nurses. Therefore, nurses must be diligent in maintaining safety awareness for not only their patients but also themselves.

Musculosketal injuries are among the most frequent physical injuries and are attributed to moving patients from the bed to the chair or stretcher, repositioning, and attempting to prevent a patient from falling (Stokowski, 2014). Additionally, repeated tasks that require bending, pushing, and pulling may also be problematic (Stokowski, 2014).

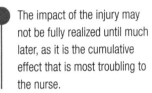 The impact of the injury may not be fully realized until much later, as it is the cumulative effect that is most troubling to the nurse.

If you have experienced a musculosketal injury, be sure to complete and submit the organization's incident report. You should also be seen by a physician or another care provider for a physical assessment to determine the extent of the injury.

To prevent further injury, follow the organization's policies and procedures for proper lifting, transferring, and moving patients. If the organization provides lift equipment, you need to use it. If you do not, get additional help when moving patients or doing any type of heavy lifting. If you have been placed on lifting restrictions, follow them for the stated length of time. Review and implement proper body mechanics for lifting.

Nurses may also be accidentally shocked by equipment and emergency resuscitation paddles, and there is the potential to be burned by using cauterization machines. Cleaning solutions and disinfectants may cause inhalation problems and exacerbate allergies.

Many nurses work in radiation therapy and therefore are at risk for radiation exposure and burns. Because radiation is invisible and odorless, there is no way to be sure of exposure. At the minimum, nurses may experience nausea, vomiting, erythema, dermatitis, and diarrhea; however, long-term exposure may cause cancer, sterilization, bone marrow suppression, congenital defects, and death (Stokowski, 2014).

Nurses working with lasers are potentially at risk for thermal injury to the skin and eyes (Stokowski, 2014). Surgical nurses are in danger of inhalation problems from toxic gases and blood-borne pathogens (Pierce, Lacey, Lippert, & Franke, 2011).

You must use caution when handling urine, stool, blood, and emesis by wearing gloves and a face shield when necessary. The Occupational Safety and Health Administration (OSHA) has developed the simplified document *Hazard Communication Standard*, providing a more common and understandable approach to categorizing chemicals and communicating hazard information. The updated document is the *Employee Right to Understand*, at https://www.osha.gov/dsg/hazcom/ghd053107.html (Stokowski, 2014). Though Stokowski points out that proper education is paramount, avoiding the chemicals when possible is preferred (2014).

Protecting Yourself

No one will protect you like you will. Be in control of your personal well-being. Know the policies on workplace violence where you work, and know how to prevent it from happening or how to report violent behaviors from others. Ensure that you are aware of the organization's policies and procedures for workplace safety. Know where to locate the information and what to do if you find faulty equipment or if you or a coworker is injured. Follow all isolation procedures and other safety precautions established in your organization. Be aware of your surroundings and of the people who are present when you are working. Most importantly, know how to protect yourself from developing a workplace injury or from being a victim of violence.

The following list gives you some ways to protect yourself:

- Wear protective gear when appropriate, such as a mask, an eye shield, gloves, shoe covers, and gown.

- Do not recap needles.

- Use needleless devices when appropriate.

- Dispose of used needles immediately into sharps containers.

- If you are moving across the room to dispose of a used syringe, hold the syringe upright in front of you to avoid sticking yourself or others.

- Engage in safety continuing education programs.

- Use adequate lighting.

- Check instrument trays for sharp spots before picking up.

- Avoid chemical exposure, wear proper protective clothing when necessary, and avoid exposure when possible.

- Minimize radiation exposure by wearing protective clothing and avoiding radiation when possible.

- Properly dispose of contaminated material.

- Complete and submit an incident report if you sustain an injury, and seek a medical assessment to substantiate the injury.

- Stop workplace violence, know your organization's policies, refrain from violent behavior, confront situations whenever possible, and report people who exhibit violent behaviors.

Healthcare organizations are complex, and many people come and go every day. Nurses are caring for patients with a variety of emotional, psychosocial, and physical illnesses. Family members may be stressed and may lack coping skills to deal with complex and emotional decisions.

Violence in healthcare organizations is among the highest in all working environments, and it impacts the safety of not only nurses but also other providers of care and our patients. Violence may come in many forms, from the not-so-obvious eye rolling and sighing to more violent behaviors such as gunshots, stabbings, and physical assaults that may result in physical and emotional injury and even death.

In addition, nurses are working with lots of different equipment, some of it heavy, bulky, and unstable and often in confined spaces. Nurses are also exposed to many different hazards such as inhalants, topical chemicals, blood-borne pathogens, diseases, high-voltage electrical equipment, and instruments that may result in puncture wounds or skin lacerations. Nurses should be aware of the many potential hazards in the workplace and opportunities for people to commit violent behaviors and then learn how to protect themselves from violence and injury.

Chapter Checkup

Key points from this chapter include:

❑ As a nurse, you will face violence, in both obvious and non-obvious ways.

❑ Recognize the many types of violent behaviors.

❑ Reduce the possibility that you become a victim of violence.

❑ Avoid workplace injuries.

❑ Protect yourself from an injury.

❑ Know what to do if you sustain an injury.

References

Canadian Centre for Occupational Health and Safety (CCOHS). (2014). Needlestick and sharps injuries. Retrieved from http://www.ccohs.ca/oshanswers/diseases/needlestick_injuries.html

Centers for Disease Control and Prevention (CDC). (2014a). Preventing needlestick injuries in healthcare settings. Retrieved from http://www.cdc.gov/niosh/docs/2000-108

Centers for Disease Control and Prevention (CDC). (2014b). Workplace safety and health topics. Retrieved from http://www.cdc.gov/niosh/topics/healthcare

Gates, D. M., Gillespie, G. L., & Succop, P. (2011). Violence against nurses and its impact on stress and productivity. *Nursing Economics, 29*(2), 59–66.

Glacki-Smith, J., Juarez, A. M., Boyett, L., Homeyer, C., Robinson, L., & Maclean, S. (2010). Violence against nurses working in U.S. emergency departments. *Journal of Nursing Administration, 39*(7–8), 340–349.

Howard, P. K., & Gilboy, N. (2009). Workplace violence. *Advanced Emergency Nursing Journal, 31*(2), 94–100.

McPhaul, K. M., & Lipscomb, J. A. (2004). Workplace violence in healthcare: Recognized but not regulated. *The Online Journal of Issues in Nursing, 93*(3). Retrieved from www.nursingworld.org/MainMenuCategories/ANAMarketplace/ANAPeriodicals/OJIN/TableofContents/Volume92004/No3Sept04/ViolenceinHealthCare.html

Nachreiner, N. M., Hansen, H. E., Okano, A., Gerberich, S. G., Ryan, A. D., McGovern, P. M., … Watt, G. D. (2007). Difference in work-related violence by nurse license type. *Journal of Professional Nursing, 23*(5), 290–300.

Nordqvist, C. (2013, July 20). Healthcare most dangerous place for workplace injuries. *Medical News Today.* Retrieved from http://www.medicalnewstoday.com/articles/263709.php

OSHA and Worker Safety Joint Commission. (2012). Environment of care news, *15*(1). Retrieved from http://www.jcrinc.com/assets/1/7/ECNews-Jan-2012.pdf

Papa, A., & Venella, J. (2013). Workplace violence in healthcare: Strategies for advocacy. *The Online Journal of Issues in Nursing, 18*(1). doi: 10.3912/OJIN.Vol18NO01Man05

Pierce, J. S., Lacey, S. E., Lippert, J. F., & Franke, J. E. (2011). Laser-generated air contaminants from medial laser applications: A state of the science review of exposure characterization, health effects, and control. *Journal of Occupational Environment Hygiene, 8*, 447–466.

Speroni, K. G., Fitch, T., Dawson, E., Dugan, L., & Atherton, M. (2013). Incidence and cost of nurse workplace violence perpetrated by hospital patients or visitors. *Journal of Emergency Nursing, 40*(3), 218–228. doi: http://dx.doi.org/10.1016/j.jen.2013.05.014

Stokowski, L. A. (2014). The risky business of nursing. Medscape Family Medicine, 2–8. Retrieved from www.medscape.com/viewarticle/818437_2

Sullivan, E. J. (2013). *Effective leadership and management in nursing* (8th ed.). Upper Saddle River, NJ: Pearson.

Thomas, C. M. (2010). Teaching nursing students and newly registered nurses strategies to deal with violent behaviors in the professional practice environment. *The Journal of Continuing Education in Nursing, 41*(7), 299–310.

Trotto, S. (2014). Workplace violence in health care. *Safety & Health.* Retrieved from http://www.safetyandhealthmagazine.com/articles/print/11172-workplace-violence-in-health-care-nurses

United States Bureau of Labor Statistics, Occupational Safety & Health Administration. (2010). Workplace violence. Retrieved from https://www.osha.gov/SLTC/healthcarefacilities/violence.html

Wood, H., & Brott, E. F. (2013). Key considerations: Healthcare workplace violence. *Pro Assurance, 6*(1), 2–7. Retrieved from www.proassurance.com/pdfindex/?guid=2a57e11c-7cc6-45fa-8c1e-b2c147a79265

9

LOOKING TO PRACTICE OUTSIDE OF THE HOSPITAL

ELEMENTS OF LOOKING TO PRACTICE OUTSIDE OF THE HOSPITAL

1. Considers the differences between practice in hospitals and practice not in hospitals
2. Examines the effects of the Affordable Care Act on nursing
3. Recognizes that a majority of RNs will work in the community
4. Acknowledges that one can be an RN while never having practiced in acute care
5. Describes how your personality impacts your preferred employment setting

As a new registered nurse (RN), most of your clinical experience and exposure to nursing has been in the acute care setting. Not surprisingly, you're likely to go directly into a hospital for your first position. The Health Resources and Services Administration (HRSA) notes that approximately 63% of RNs work in the acute care setting (HRSA, 2013), which includes direct care RNs and administrative RN staff.

Employment of registered nurses is projected to grow 19% from 2012 to 2022, faster than the average for all occupations. This growth will occur for a number of reasons, including an increased emphasis on preventive care (Bureau of Labor Statistics, 2015), driven now by healthcare reform. In this chapter, we will touch on various options for practicing as an RN, even as a new RN, outside the hospital setting.

The World of Opportunities Outside the Acute Care Environment

Because much of your experience to date was in the hospital setting, you, like most new nurses, may have decided on specific service lines to apply for or submitted an application already. Additionally, you may have been told to go get hospital experience first and then go into the community to work. Most of the time, this advice comes from someone who has never worked in the community setting.

 Determine the best path for yourself. You may want to choose the hospital setting while others go directly into the community setting.

Nurses, and nursing care, which was mostly in the community more than 100 years ago, moved into hospitals around the time of the Great Depression. This move was made due to decreased funding for public health and the lessened ability of private families to afford private nursing care, which made hospitals a more stable source of income for nurses.

A lot has changed since then, and we have come full circle back to the community. We will talk more about nonhospital positions later, but first we will describe the distribution of the RN workforce, workforce projections, and the Patient Protection and Affordable Care Act. All these elements are important in shaping healthcare reform and where employment will be in the future.

> Choose with purpose the setting in which you will practice. Do not get into a position where you burn out quickly or your personality doesn't match up well with the patient/care interactions. And do not assimilate into this new position by viewing it as "just work," clocking in and out and waiting for your time off each week. This method will bring you a life of meaningless work and time lost—your time. It may also lead to early burnout and job dissatisfaction.

Hospitals and Acute Care Setting

Working in a hospital definitely now has perceived benefits. *Perceived benefits* typically include higher starting pay, shift differentials, and those 12-hour shifts, giving you 4 days off a week. Because patients in hospitals need round-the-clock care, nurses in these settings usually work in rotating shifts, covering all 24 hours. You may work nights, weekends, and holidays in addition to being on call.

Unlike hospital nurses, those who work in the community (and in offices, schools, and other locations that do not provide 24-hour care) are more likely to work regular business hours (Bureau of Labor Statistics, 2015). Though 12-hour shifts with 4 days off seems like a good lifestyle choice, it can create a hardship for those with children, caregiving responsibilities, and families. It may also interfere with sleep patterns and overall physical and emotional health.

As noted earlier in this chapter, not all RNs work in hospitals. Nurses work in just about any area one can imagine (see Table 9.1), and in any area that has yet to be thought up. As healthcare reform continues, this distribution will change, and more nurses will need to go into community-based employment, as nursing positions shift from acute care to community and public health.

Table 9.1   Distribution of RN Workforce in the United States

Setting	Urban	Rural	All
Hospital	63.9	59.4	63.2
Nursing Care Facility	6.8	10.6	7.4
Office of Physician	4.8	4.5	4.8
Home Healthcare Service	3.6	4.6	3.8
Outpatient Care Center	4.5	5.3	4.6
Other Healthcare Service	5.6	4.6	5.4
Elementary and Secondary School	2.2	2.3	2.2
Employment Service	2.1	1.9	2.1
Insurance Carrier	1.0	0.3	0.9
Administration of HR Program	1.2	2.2	1.4
Justice, Public Order, and Safety	0.5	1.3	0.6
Office of Other Practitioner	0.3	0.2	0.3
College or University	0.6	0.4	0.6
Residential Facility, w/o Nursing	0.3	0.5	0.4
All Other	2.6	2.2	2.5
Total	100	100	100

(HRSA, 2013)

Healthcare reform is a major player in determining nursing workforce needs. Before the passage of the Patient Protection and

Affordable Care Act (PPACA) on March 23, 2010, projections (see Table 9.2) demonstrated a growing need for community nurses. With the passage of PPACA, these projections will increase in need.

Table 9.2   The Department of Labor's Employment Increases between 2006–2016 per Nurse Employer Type

Increase	Nurse Employer
25%	Offices of physicians
23%	Home healthcare services
34%	Outpatient care centers, except mental health and substance abuse
33%	Employment services
23%	General medical and surgical hospitals, public and private
23%	Nursing care facilities

Patient Protection and Affordable Care Act

If you haven't heard about the Patient Protection and Affordable Care Act (PPACA), undoubtedly you have heard about Obama-Care. It is one and the same, and it is healthcare reform. Though this act does not constitute total reform, it is partial reform that is nudging the United States away from a system that is not feasible to continue in its current form. Figure 9.1 demonstrates what we in the United States spend on healthcare compared to what we spend on education and defense.

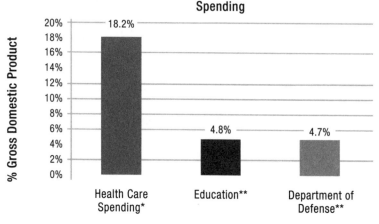

Figure 9.1   Comparison of Spending by Percentage of GDP
(Mensik, 2013)

Furthermore, the Institute of Medicine (IOM, 2012) reported that healthcare waste equals $750 billion annually. How large is $750 billion? The 1-year estimate of healthcare waste is equal to more than 10 years of Medicare cuts in President Obama's healthcare law, or, put another way, more than the Department of Defense budget or more than enough to care for the uninsured (IOM, 2012).

So, what does this information have to do with you and working outside the hospital? It directly affects the need for nurses and where nurses are needed. The shift in healthcare settings to focus on less costly preventive care and move away from sick care (hospital care) will produce an increased or expanded role for:

1. Preventive care

2. Nurse practitioners

3. Patient education

RNs and advanced practice registered nurses (APRNs) play a major role in decreasing costs and reforming the U.S. healthcare system. Additionally, major pieces of the PPACA are in place, with only a few more pieces finalizing into place through 2018. The biggest changes in the PPACA include:

- Lifetime maximums are now a thing of the past.

- Insurance companies can no longer drop coverage for individuals who become ill.

- There are no more annual limits, benefiting those with catastrophic illness.

- Children up to age 26 can remain on their parent's plan.

- Small businesses offering insurance can apply for a 35% tax credit for premiums paid.

- New plans written going forward must offer preventive care with no co-pays or deductibles.

- Medicare Part D participants will receive a $250 credit to help with the "doughnut hole," or coverage gap.

- Retirees aged 55–64 will be offered access to a reinsurance program.

- No one can be denied insurance for preexisting conditions.

- The federally subsidized, high-risk pools established in 2010 will be, and states will be, required to have their insurance exchanges in place.

- Annual caps on benefits are banned completely.

- All plans offer preventive care without co-pays or deductibles.

Many of you will eventually, if not at first, be employed in a community or public health setting. Through your clinical rotations, you may have been initially exposed to some of these settings, depending on your program.

 If you want to learn more about PPACA and its impact, see one of the many great resources on the Internet, including the Kaiser Family Foundation website: http://kff.org/topic/health-reform

Ambulatory Care

Many settings of care are also specialty types of nursing care. *Ambulatory* is a specialty nursing practice, for example. The American Academy of Ambulatory Care Nursing (AAACN) notes many facets that make up ambulatory care nursing. Clinics, urgent care, telehealth, and surgical centers are some of the usual settings and modes of care provided in the ambulatory setting. The RN/patient encounter may occur once or as a series of occurrences. These occurrences usually last fewer than 24 hours, and they occur singly or in group settings (AAACN, 2015).

For more information, consider visiting the AAACN website at https://www.aaacn.org/what-ambulatory-care-nursing

The RN in ambulatory care:

- Promotes optimal wellness
- Participates in the management of acute illness
- Assists the patient in managing the effects of chronic disease and disability
- Provides support in end-of-life care (AAACN, 2015)

Quite often, care is provided across the life span to individuals, families, caregivers, groups, populations, and communities (AAACN, 2015).

Public Health

Public health is the practice of promoting and protecting the health of populations. The primary focus is not on providing direct care to individuals in a community setting but rather on promoting, assessing, and ensuring the health of the entire population.

Types of community services that public health nurses provide include:

- Clinical services

- Communicable disease surveillance and outreach

- Immunizations

- Health education programs

- Policy promotion

- Development of emergency response plans and actions

- Public health emergencies around the nation

- Work on research, policy, and regulation

- Work in tribal clinics, immigration detention centers, and federal prisons

Nurses working in public health may be commissioned and civil employees (USPHS, 2015).

The U.S. public health system (PHS) is under the direction of the U.S. Department of Health and Human Services (HHS). Within the U.S. public health system is the Nursing Professional Advisory Committee (N-PAC), composed of nursing representatives (both civil service and Commissioned Corps). This committee provides advice and consultation to the surgeon general of the United States (SG), to the PHS chief nurse officer (CNO), and to HHS, federal health, and other leadership (such as HHS agency/program heads and other federal agencies and programs that utilize PHS nursing personnel) (USPHS, 2015).

To learn more about public health, visit the following websites:

Association of Public Health Nurses at http://phnurse.org

U.S. Public Health Service Nursing at http://phs-nurse.org/welcome

Home Health

The purpose of home health nursing is to restore and maintain a patient's maximal level of function and health. These services are rendered in lieu of hospitalization or confinement in an extended care facility or ambulatory care setting. Many people interchange home healthcare with home care. However, *home care* is typically noted as the wide range of services that include home medical/durable equipment, home infusion therapy, and private (not skilled nursing) home care. *Home healthcare* (or *home health nursing*) refers to services provided in a person's home setting that require the skills of an RN or a physical therapist or speech therapist. Insurance companies will pay for skilled home services, but they do not pay for private home care services that are typically custodial and include activities such as housekeeping and cooking. Custodial care does not require the skills of an RN. However, as will be discussed later in the chapter content on private duty nursing, it may include nonskilled functions.

Home health nursing requires that you can function autonomously and can drive to multiple patients' homes during the day. Your interaction with other team members might be during joint home health visits or phone calls and emails to your nurse manager in the office.

Home health nursing is not for everyone. Whereas in the hospital a patient is in your setting for care, in this scenario you are in the patient's setting. Patient interaction is usually different because the person is more relaxed in familiar surroundings.

Typically, home health RNs are also case managers. These case managers are different from those in the hospital such that they provide direct patient care. In addition to managing a wound or evaluating symptoms, the RN ensures that orders are in place, manages other nursing staff visits, and requests from insurance companies any updates and approvals for continuing visits.

A home health RN's caseload may be anywhere from 20 to 40 patients, with an average of 25 to 30. The RN does not see each patient every day, as different patient needs vary, but the RN manages the patient needs with visit frequencies within a care team for that patient. Team members vary patient-to-patient based on needs, but all home health agencies must provide, at minimum, physical, occupational, and speech therapists and RN, social work, and nursing assistant services.

As a former home health nurse myself, I have visited every type of home, from multimillion-dollar mansions to a bug-infested mobile home, all in the same day. As the nurse, you are recognized as a guest in the patient's home, and you need to be truly nonjudgmental and honor the choice for how each person lives. I loved being a home health nurse for the variety and independence.

To learn more about home health nursing, visit the Home Healthcare Nurses Association website for more information: www.hhna.org

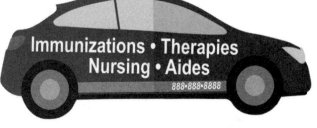

Hospice

Hospice care is similar to home healthcare in that you visit people in their home environments: a house, a nursing home, or an assisted living apartment, for example. However, unlike home healthcare, where the goal is to maintain and restore health, the goal of *hospice care* is to maintain or improve quality of life for someone whose illness, disease, or condition is unlikely to be cured (Hospice Foundation of America, 2015). Typically, hospice patients have cancer, but many hospice patients may be admitted to services for late-stage heart, lung, or kidney disease, or advanced Alzheimer's disease or dementia. Hospice was once exclusively for adults, but many hospice programs now accept infants, children, and adolescents.

As in home health, RNs function like case managers but may be called *team leaders*. Due to the intense nature of end of life, with patient and family interactions, a hospice RN's typical caseload may be between 8 and 14 patients. Typical team members include a nursing assistant, a physician or nurse practitioner, social worker, and chaplain. End-of-life care is rewarding but not for everyone. The goal of hospice care is to also have people die at home and not in a hospital. However, depending on symptom management, such as severe pain, people may be admitted to an in-patient hospice house for care.

 You can find the Hospice and Palliative Care Nurses Association website at http://hpna.advancingexpertcare.org

Long-Term Care

A *long-term care nurse* cares for patients who have a disability or an illness and are in need of extended care. Care is typically provided in nursing homes, assisted living residences, continuing care retirement communities, rehabilitation centers, and home- and community-based programs. In these settings, the RN will provide care to the elderly and younger patients with disabilities. Depending on the setting, the RN's responsibilities will vary, from charge nurse and then team leader to staff RN. Frequently in these settings there are fewer and fewer RNs and more licensed practical nurses (LPNs) and assistive personnel such as nursing assistants.

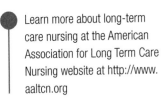 Learn more about long-term care nursing at the American Association for Long Term Care Nursing website at http://www.aaltcn.org

EXPERIENCE FROM THE FIELD: THE BURGUNDY BOX

They say all good things come in small packages. That was the burgundy box. I met Phillip (Phil) Davis on a hot summer day in a secured dementia unit. He had a quiet demeanor and would often sit and gaze out the window as though he were consumed with the world's emotions. They say friendship often strikes at the most inopportune time. Well, this was that time. He glanced at me with a sad look, as though the weight of the world were on his shoulders, and that is the moment we became friends.

It was 3 years later, around the holidays after Phil passed away, when I first reached for the burgundy box. Like fine red wine, the box symbolized what was left of the memories of Phil. Birth pictures, college pictures, service pictures, wife, girlfriend, sister, and who was the tall, thin man I had met in the dementia unit and become friends with, I wondered. He had once been an intelligent, charming person. Because of his illness, he had become forgetful and started having auditory and visual hallucinations. It was then I found out that end-stage pancreatic cancer had metastasized to his brain. There was so much he told me during his lucid phases and so much I was left to ponder. I was determined to put the pieces together and to honor the memory and legacy of Phil.

The ward would get awfully hot in the summertime, and every day I was tasked with taking care of Phil. He was assigned to me as a patient. I sat and listened by the edge of his bed and brought him ice chips to chew on. He told me he had been born in Bellevue, Washington, in the early 1950s. He was from an affluent neighborhood. He spoke about the evergreens and the state parks and dreamed of going into the Navy. Like any other child, he'd had a normal childhood where he laughed and played and developed a passion for aircraft, yet at the same time experienced a strict upbringing. His days had been filled with music lessons, art lessons, baseball, reading, and math. Having no time to himself, Phil had been forced to grow up rather fast. Soon after, his sister was born. From this moment, he developed a close-yet-jealous type of relationship with his sister. After being an only child for so long, having to share the spotlight wasn't something Phil adapted to quickly. He dreamed of the days he could leave home and join the Naval Academy.

Phil had attended the Army and Navy Academy in Carlsbad, California, and after high school had joined the Army. He'd had a close relationship with his family and sent weekly letters updating his parents on his status. He graduated from the military academy in 1972 and went on to have a seemingly full career. After their mother died in 1983, his sister, Sharon Davis, convinced him to move to Arizona to rekindle their relationship. Phil never shared with me the demise of the relationship in the 1970s. He did share about the wonderful moments of when his sister opened his eyes to a new world and introduced him to his wife. He was married only 1 year when he and his wife welcomed their daughter. Sitting on the floor looking at the burgundy box, I remembered his love for his daughter.

Although Phil had known that he had only a few weeks or months to live, he spoke about all the things he still wanted to do with his life. Phil never asked for anything. One day, Timothy Abbruscato, one of the nurses from the unit, told me that Phil loved blueberry yogurt. From then on, I always asked him whether he wanted to eat any other foods. He would say that he simply wanted blueberry yogurt. I brought him the blueberry yogurt.

During the holidays, Phil was heavily involved with decorating the facility. He often described his upbringing around the holidays. He had found that a lot of the holidays were spent at the homes of the friends he had met in the academy. He missed feeling the closeness of his family. Timothy tried for months to get in touch with Phil's family before his final days set in.

Phil died one sunny afternoon with Timothy by his side. He was cremated. He died alone. I often think about Phil and the memories we shared. Anyone who has lost a close friend knows the pain that accompanies it. Every year around the holidays, I take some time to honor the memory of Phil. I even eat some blueberry yogurt. I remember the simple pleasures in life. For at the end of life's journey, if all we have is a burgundy box, I want to make sure that the box is filled with love, joy, and memories, in the spirit of Phil.

Long-term care provides nurses with the opportunity to build relationships, unlike in the acute care setting with its short patient admissions. If you enjoy developing relationships with others, this setting will give you the ability to build relationships with residents as you provide a caring environment for them over months and years.

—Brenda Geisler, MSN, FNP-C, and Ana Tackett

School Nursing

In the late 1800s Lillian Wald founded school nursing after experiencing success in public health (Zaiger, 2006). In the 1900s, school nurses focused primarily on communicable diseases (NASN, 2011). It was around this time that a small group of nurses came together to establish the Lillian Wald Henry Street Settlement (Vessey & McGowan, 2006). Over the years the issues expanded to include chronic conditions such as diabetes, asthma, and obesity.

Now 70,000 school nurses work in the United States (HRSA, 2010). School nurses, who are responsible for elementary schoolchildren through high school students, take care of a wide variety of healthcare and developmental needs. School nurses provide nursing care, apply treatments, and administer medication. In addition, they are responsible for maintaining school health records including immunization and vaccination records.

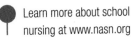 Learn more about school nursing at www.nasn.org

Determining Where You Fit Best

Though little research exists to help you decide where you should work after nursing school, you have a few points to consider. Many new RNs change positions after their first year, and the reasons vary, including not realizing that they dislike a unit or service type until they've spent a few months there. Though you need to follow your heart, think about your own personality and how you may or may not fit with the specifics of a unit. Answer these questions:

1. Do you like to build relationships and interact with patients? An outpatient setting that allows you more time to interact and build relationships, such as in long-term care, might be best for you.

2. Are you a multitasker? The medical surgical unit is the choice for you. You will see different types of patients with different needs, utilizing your skills to multitask.

3. Do you prefer to manage one or two patients at a time, and do you have technical skills? Try the OR or ICU.

4. Do you like quick-paced work and adrenaline? The emergency department is likely a good spot for you.

5. Do you like planning and organizing large-scale events and processes? Public health might work for you.

6. Do you prefer to get to know your patients on a more personal level? Try home care.

7. Do you like the elderly? Consider long-term care or assistive living communities.

8. Are you drawn to help people die with dignity? Then hospice might be a rewarding career option.

9. Do you like to work with children but also want holidays and summers free? Consider school nursing.

10. Do you like to work with all people regarding wellness but do not want to work in a hospital? Give parish nursing a try.

Though this is a quick list, it doesn't mean that you don't build relationships in all areas or multitask or provide technically complex care to patients in all areas. Each department, area, or service line has a unique patient population and ways that patients are cared for and managed. Take these unique characteristics into consideration when you are looking for the best match with your personality. We want you to be happy with your new position and grow into an amazing professional RN.

These are just some of the many settings for employment after you graduate. A world of possibilities lies outside the hospital setting. Whether you go to the hospital first or go directly into a nonhospital setting, you will never be bored in your nursing career. And, after healthcare reform and PPACA, more and more nursing care will be provided in community settings.

Chapter Checkup

Key points from this chapter include:

❑ In deciding which setting to work in, you need to determine the best path for yourself. Not everyone fits into a hospital setting, and not everyone likes ambulatory care.

❑ As healthcare reform continues, this distribution will change, and more nurses will need to go into community-based employment.

❑ Almost 40% of nurses do not work in an acute care setting. Think outside of the box—the hospital box, that is.

References

American Academy of Ambulatory Care Nursing (AAACN). (2015). What is ambulatory care nursing? Retrieved from https://www.aaacn.org/what-ambulatory-care-nursing

Bureau of Labor Statistics, U.S. Department of Labor. (2015). *Occupational outlook handbook*. Registered nurses. Retrieved from http://www.bls.gov/ooh/healthcare/registered-nurses.htm

Health Resources and Services Administration (HRSA). (2010). Retrieved from http://bhpr.hrsa.gov/healthworkforce/rnsurveys/rnsurveyinitial2008.pdf

Health Resources and Services Administration (HRSA). (2013). The U.S. nursing workforce: Trends in supply and education. Bureau of Health Professions. National Center for Health Workforce Analysis. Retrieved from http://bhpr.hrsa.gov/healthworkforce/reports/nursingworkforce/nursingworkforcefullreport.pdf

Hospice Foundation of America. (2015). What is hospice? Retrieved from http://hospicefoundation.org/End-of-Life-Support-and-Resources/Coping-with-Terminal-Illness/Hospice-Services

Institute of Medicine (IOM). (2012). Best care at lower cost: The path to continuously learning healthcare in America. Committee on the Learning Health Care System in America. Smith, M., Saunders, R., Stuckhardt, L., & McGinnis, J. M. (Eds.). Washington, DC: The National Academies Press.

Mensik, J. (2013). *The nurse manager's guide to innovative staffing*. Indianapolis, IN: Sigma Theta Tau International.

National Association of School Nurses (NASN). (2011). Position statement: Role of the school nurse. Silver Spring, MD: Author.

National Coalition on Health Care. (2011). Quick facts. Washington, DC. Retrieved from http://nchc.org/facts-resources/quick-facts

Nursing in the United States. (2015). Wikipedia. Retrieved from http://en.wikipedia.org/wiki/Nursing_in_the_United_States

United States Department of Defense Fiscal Year 2013 Budget Request (2012). Office of the Under Secretary of Defense (Comptroller)/Chief Financial Officer. Retrieved from http://comptroller.defense.gov/budget.html

U.S. Public Health Service (USPHS). (2015). USPHS Nursing. Retrieved from http://phs-nurse.org/welcome

Vessey, J. A., & McGowan, K. A. (2006). A successful public health experiment: School nursing. *Pediatric Nurse, 32*(3), 255–256.

Zaiger, D. S. (2006). Historical perspectives of school nursing. *School nursing: A comprehensive text*, pp. 3–24. Philadelphia, PA: F.A. Davis Company.

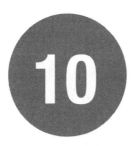

CONTINUING EDUCATION AND ADVANCED DEGREES

ELEMENTS OF CONTINUING EDUCATION AND ADVANCED DEGREES

1. Identifies the different types of nursing degree programs

2. Emphasizes the BSN as the entry-level degree

3. Offers real-life personal stories about nursing degree paths

4. Discusses advanced degrees such as the master's, post master's certificate programs, and doctorate in nursing and related fields

5. Examines a variety of continuing education options

6. Stresses the importance of nursing organizations

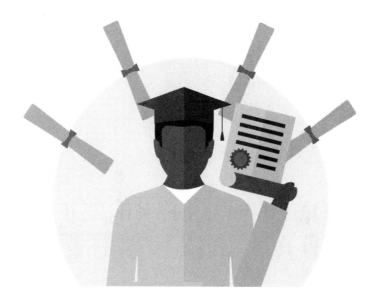

Healthcare is in a constant state of change. This constant change makes it necessary for nurses to remain knowledgeable, via lifelong learning, about the current best practice. Nurses have many options to continue their education, including degreed and non-degreed programs and self-study in continuing education programs (CE). The first part of this chapter takes a serious look at the benefits of each degree. Then the rest of the chapter looks at continuing education options.

Associate Degree (ASN/ADN)

The ASN/ADN provides an excellent foundation on which many registered nurses (RNs) begin professional practice. Nurses prepared at the associate degree level are considered *generalist;* this degree requires courses that provide general nursing experience. For example, these general courses are similar to the baccalaureate degree, including the foundation courses of pathophysiology, anatomy and physiology, fundamentals in nursing, physical assessment, medical surgical nursing, maternal health, pediatrics, mental health, and pharmacology. However, the associate degree does not include nursing management and leadership, research, community health, or statistics.

Though it is true that the associate-degreed nurse sits for the same NCLEX exam, the baccalaureate-prepared nurse practices at a much broader level and may have a better interpretation of the cultural, political, economic, and social issues now facing patients and influencing healthcare delivery (Rosseter, 2015). It is evident the RN's role has become much more complex and increasingly requires the educational background of the baccalaureate degree. Because of the increase in nursing demands, in some states, like Indiana, hospitals are requiring RNs to have their baccalaureate degrees completed in a certain time frame (e.g., 2015).

The Baccalaureate Degree (BSN)

The Robert Wood Johnson Foundation initiated the report *The Future of Nursing: Leading Change, Advancing Health* to increase the number of baccalaureate-prepared nurses up to 80% by 2020 (IOM, 2010). In addition, Patricia Benner and a team of researchers published a study, *Educating Nurses: A Call for Radical Transformation*, recommending that the baccalaureate degree be the entry level for practice and that all RNs earn a master's degree within 10 years of the initial licensure (Benner, Sutphen, Leonard, & Day, 2009).

There is much debate about entry level and advanced degrees for registered nurses. In 2003 the National Council of State Boards of Nursing explored this topic, and it still continues to be debated (AACN, 2012; Smith, 2003). The American Association of Colleges of Nursing (AACN) identifies the baccalaureate degree (BSN) as preparing the nurse to meet the rigorous demands placed on today's nurses (AACN, 2015). The BSN nurse has a strong foundation in leadership, critical thinking, problem solving, case management, and health promotion (AACN, 2015). The AACN strongly advocates for the BSN-prepared nurse, while encouraging healthcare organizations to endorse an environment that embraces lifelong learning and proposes incentives for registered nurses to earn baccalaureate and higher degrees. The BSN-prepared nurse has a broader scope of practice, providing a more comprehensive understanding of cultural, political, social, diversity, and economic issues impacting clients and influencing healthcare delivery (AACN, 2015).

The Health Resources and Services Administration (HRSA) released a report indicating that only 55% of all nurses in the United States had earned a baccalaureate degree or higher (HRSA, 2013). The National Advisory Council on Nurse Education and Practice (NACNEP) urged that two-thirds (67%) of all nurses should earn, at minimum, a baccalaureate or advanced degree (HRSA, 2013). As you can see, there is still a deficit between the number of baccalaureate-prepared RNs that HRSA reports and the number encouraged by NACNEP.

Why the BSN?

Rosseter (2015) indicates that the liberal arts classes included in a baccalaureate plan of study help prepare a better nurse. Liberal art courses develop a sense of analytical and creative thinking. These types of analytical skills are useful when using evidence-based practice (EBP). BSN-prepared nurses appear to be more effective, and stronger, in the areas of communication, assessment, cultural sensitivity, and resourcefulness (Rosseter, 2015). The baccalaureate-prepared nurse has many more career options than an associate-prepared nurse, and employers are seeking RNs with a baccalaureate degree and higher (Xu, 2013).

You can earn a baccalaureate degree in several ways, such as the traditional 4-year college program, an RN-to-BSN transition program, or an LPN-to-RN program. These programs build on the associate degree foundation, and in most programs completion takes only 18–24 months. Many RN-to-BSN programs are conveniently offered in the evenings at places of employment, in online classes, and in the traditional classroom setting. Many employers are willing to help pay for the cost for nurses to return to college for additional degrees.

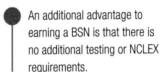 An additional advantage to earning a BSN is that there is no additional testing or NCLEX requirements.

EXPERIENCE FROM THE FIELD: CONTINUING EDUCATION AND ADVANCED DEGREES

When I graduated from my BSN program, I knew that I wanted to get my master's degree in nursing education. Many faculty inspired me to pass on the knowledge and passion I have for nursing, and many people questioned whether I should go right away or gain more experience and advance down my career path. I had such a burning desire to teach that I decided to jump in with both feet one year after my first graduation.

I was blessed to be accepted into a master's cohort, which was one of the best things to happen at this point in my career. One important piece of advice for attending grad school is to find the format and the type of program that works best for you. For me, having a mainly in-person, ground program was what helped engage me in the material and the dialogue, and continued to build my passion for nursing. If you end up in a program that does not work for you, you will resent it, and it will not fulfill your desire for furthering your education.

Many programs for advanced degrees are out there, so take the time to find the right fit for you. Nursing needs people who are willing to advance their educations for their patients, coworkers, populations, and, ultimately, profession, so follow your heart and reach for the sky.

–Jennifer Tucker, MA, RN

Master's Degree

After you have earned a baccalaureate degree, you may want to start thinking about earning a master's degree. There are many different track options for nurses seeking a master's degree, such as nurse educator, clinical nurse leader, nurse administrator, nurse practitioner, nurse researcher, and clinical nurse specialist. More than 500 schools of nursing in the United States offer more than 2,000 different graduate programs (AACN, 2014).

Many programs require students to pass the graduate record exam (GRE) to be admitted to the program; however, many university programs do not require the GRE.

DID YOU KNOW?

The GRE is a graduate admission exam with a general exam and seven subject areas that can be tested, including microbiology, biology, chemistry, mathematics, psychology, English, and physics (www.ets.org/gre).

Entry-level master's degree programs will generally take 2–3 years for completion if you are entering the program with a baccalaureate degree. On completion of a master's program, you will be granted a master of science in nursing (MSN), master of science (MS), or master of nursing (MN) depending on the individual university degree requirements.

RN-to-master's degree programs were created for nurses who have earned associate degrees. Many of these programs may take only 2–3 years to accomplish and may be pursued in a traditional classroom and/or online. These programs are growing in popularity and have increased over the past 20 years (AACN, 2014a). Nurses interested in a specific area of practice often consider a dual master's program. Some of these programs combine nursing with business, public, or health administration (AACN, 2014b).

Post Master's Certificate

Another option for continuing education is the post master's certificate programs. The certificate programs are for nurses who have already earned a master's degree but want to extend their education to other areas of interest such as education, administration, gerontology, family nurse practitioner, palliative care, and nursing informatics (AACN, 2014). The amount of time to complete the certificate program will most often depend on the specific area of interest, but most certificate programs are intended to be completed within 1–2 years.

Doctoral Degree

The doctoral degree is considered the terminal degree for nurses. There are several doctoral degrees such as doctor of education (EdD), doctor of nursing practice (DNP), and doctor of philosophy (PhD).

- The *EdD* is a teaching doctorate; however, many nurse educators conduct independent research.

- The *PhD* or doctor of philosophy is considered a research doctorate, but as with the EdD, many researchers also teach.

- The *DNP* is a practice doctorate that supports the doctoral-prepared nurse practitioner in independent practice. Some DNP-prepared nurses are engaged in teaching.

Doctoral degree programs are offered in the traditional classroom environment and online. You should expect to devote 2–4 years to complete a doctoral program, depending on the specific program and number of classes taken at a given time. It is not unusual for nurses to work full time while attending classes part time. Doctoral-prepared nurses are considered experts in their fields of practice.

If you are considering earning an additional degree, ask yourself these questions:

- How committed am I to completing the program?

- Is this the best time for me to return to college?

- Do I need financial aid?

- Is my family supportive of me returning to college?

- Does my employer support my return to college?

- Do I need to work while attending college?

- How will returning to college change my schedule?

- What types of adjustments, or sacrifices, am I going to have to make when returning to college?

- Is a traditional classroom my preferred method of attendance, or will an online or hybrid (combination of both) class work better for me?

- Do I need official transcripts from my previous colleges? If so, how do I obtain these and what are the costs related to obtaining them?

- Does the college or university require a GRE or an MAT exam?

- If admission requires previous course syllabi, how do I obtain these?

Advanced practice programs are rewarding and prepare you for additional career options; however, they are rigorous, and they take time and financial and personal commitment. If you are considering an advanced practice program, consider the answers to these questions:

- What is the time commitment?

- What is the financial cost?

- Are scholarships or grants available?

- Are there clinical or practicum requirements?

- Is the coursework flexible?

- Is the program full time or part time?

- Is there a residency requirement?

- Why am I considering an advanced degree?

Save your college course syllabi, and save your sealed college transcripts. These items are crucial when you're seeking to return to college for additional degrees, and they make the admission process easier.

Nursing accrediting bodies require schools of nursing to provide very specific course content within an advanced nursing curriculum. This ensures that the student will have the course content required to take certificate exams or sit for advanced practice nursing exams. Keeping undergraduate syllabi and transcripts will verify to colleges/universities that these courses were successfully completed, with the required content.

Also note, most colleges/universities require a "C" or better in a beginning undergraduate statistics and research course for admission into a graduate program.

Continuing Education

After you have graduated from an accredited nursing program, you must engage in continuing education. Continuing education should be an ongoing process as long as you are working as a nurse. Healthcare practices are changing rapidly, and it may be difficult to keep up with the pace. To maintain competence in nursing practice, comply with laws and regulations, maintain your license, and advance your career, you must participate in continuing education (ANA, 2011). Most continuing education courses are peer reviewed and should be above the knowledge level of the initial licensure. Continuing education studies and programs do not lead to degrees. You have many opportunities to advance your education with little time and financial cost. As with all things, you must be committed.

Nursing Journals

A nursing journal is a useful source of information. You can find hundreds of nursing and related journals that are peer and non-peer reviewed. Peer reviewed journal articles have undergone a rigorous review by two to three knowledgeable nurse peers for evaluation of quality, accuracy, validity, and rigor of the manuscript prior to acceptance (Lloyd Sealy Library, 2015). Peer reviewed journals present information from nurse-led research, how-to-do-it articles, and quality improvement articles. Peer reviewed journals are excellent resources for registered nurses to learn about new and upcoming best practice strategies and current research and to help maintain competency in their area of nursing practice.

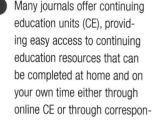

Many journals offer continuing education units (CE), providing easy access to continuing education resources that can be completed at home and on your own time either through online CE or through correspondence CE.

Online Continuing Education Websites

If you do not relish the idea of spending several days away from home at a conference or you do not like or have the time to read nursing journals, another option for learning opportunities is an online website for continuing education. Many excellent sites offer current continuing education opportunities such as MyFreeCE (www.myfreece.com), Nurse.com (www.nurse.com), and NursingWorld (nursingworld. org). These sites generally require the user to pay a fee for each CE offering or a flat rate for unlimited CE offerings within a year. Some free CE opportunities are also offered.

 You may consider writing and submitting your own CE manuscripts for potential nonreferred publication. It is a helpful way to learn and remain current in nursing practice on your own time.

Conferences

Many professional nursing conferences, in every type of specialty, are offered at the state, national, and international level. Conferences are unique in that they offer many different topics over a period of 2–4 days. Conference presenters are nursing experts who want to share research findings and evidence-based practice (EBP) in various aspects of nursing practice. A conference is a great way to connect with fellow professionals and network with others sharing similar interests. You might even want to consider being a conference presenter.

Nursing Organizations

Many nursing organizations, such as the National League for Nursing (NLN), American Nurses Association (ANA), Sigma

Theta Tau International (STTI), Emergency Nurses Association (ENA), and American Association of Critical-Care Nurses (AACN) to name a few (see the "Nursing Organizations" sidebar), offer wonderful benefits such as journals, conferences, and continuing education opportunities. Join a nursing organization that supports your areas of nursing practice, because nursing organizations also serve as a network for nurses who have interest or work in a specific area of healthcare.

NURSING ORGANIZATIONS

American Association of Critical-Care Nurses—Deals with the care of the acute critically ill patient; http://www.aacn.org

American Nurses Association—Advancement of the nursing profession; http://www.nursingworld.org

Emergency Nurses Association—Promotes safe emergency practice world-wide; https://www.ena.org/Pages/default.aspx

National League for Nursing—Devoted to excellence in nursing; http://www.nln.org

Sigma Theta Tau International—Dedicated to promoting professional development through leadership and scholarship worldwide; www.nursingsociety.org

Nurses who have been out of college and working for many years may find out that their salaries have reached the highest level offered by the employer and that those opportunities for advancement are limited or non-existent. As a result, many organizations have developed clinical or career ladders. The American Association of Colleges of Nursing endorses the career ladder concept for nurses to advance their education and improve clinical competence and quality patient care (AACN, 2010). A career ladder requires that the nurse perform specific tasks or earn additional degrees to move up the ladder. These tasks might include being on a task force or committee, serving as a preceptor or mentor, participating in EBP research, giving presentations at a conference, or earning a BSN, an MS, or a doctoral degree (Donley & Flaherty, 2008). As the nurse completes the required task, a new title is often given along with a salary increase.

Because nursing is an evidence-based practice (EBP) profession, lifelong learning is a foregone conclusion. Learning can come in many forms. Reading new research studies, subscribing to journals, and participating in continuing education are easy "at home" ways to broaden nursing knowledge. Attending conferences, actively participating in nursing conferences/workshops, and furthering education through advanced degrees are also options.

Chapter Checkup

Key points from this chapter include:

- ❏ You must engage in continuing education to remain current in practice.
- ❏ Some states require annual continuing education units as license renewal requirements. Check your state nurse practice act for further information.
- ❏ Continuing education may be formal (degree) or informal (continuing education hours).
- ❏ Many nursing organizations offer continuing education hours for free or a small fee.
- ❏ Many advanced degree programs can meet lifestyle needs.
- ❏ Read, read, read nursing journals to help stay engaged in current best practice and research.
- ❏ Consider attending a nursing conference; it is a great way to meet new people and learn.

References

American Association of Colleges of Nursing (AACN). (2010). Your nursing career: Let's look at the facts. Retrieved from http://www.aacn.nche.edu/students/your-nursing-career/facts

American Association of Colleges of Nursing (AACN). (2014a). Fact sheet: Degree completion programs for registered nurses: RN to master's degree and RN to baccalaureate programs. Retrieved from www.aacn.nche.edu/media-relations/DegreeComp.pdf

American Association of Colleges of Nursing (AACN). (2014b). Your guide to graduate nursing programs. Retrieved from www.aacn.nche.edu/publications/brochures/GradStudentsBrochure.pdf

American Association of Critical-Care Nurses (AACN). (2015). Home page. Retrieved from http://www.aacn.org

American Nurses Association (ANA). (2011). ANA nurse CE continuing education. Retrieved from http://ananursece.healthstream.com

American Nurses Credentialing Center (ANCC). (2012). The value of accreditation for continuing nursing education: Quality education contributing to quality outcomes. Retrieved from http://www.nursecredentialing.org/Accreditation/ResourcesServices/Accreditation-WhitePaper2012.pdf

Benner, P., Sutphen, M., Leonard, V., & Day, L. (2009). *Educating nurses: A call for radical transformation.* Carnegie Foundation for the Advancement of Teaching. San Francisco, CA: Jossey-Bass.

Donley, Sister R., and Flaherty, Sister M. J. (2008). Promoting professional development: Three phases of articulation in nursing education and practice. *The Online Journal of Issues in Nursing, 13*(3), Manuscript 2.

Emergency Nurses Association (ENA). (2015). Retrieved from http://www.ena.org/Pages/default.aspx

Health Resources and Services Administration (HRSA), National Center for Health Workforce Analysis. (2013). *The U. S. nursing workforce: Trends in supply and education.* Retrieved from http://bhpr.hrsa.gov/healthworkforce/supplydemand/nursing/nursingworkforce/

Institute of Medicine (IOM). (2010). *The future of nursing: Leading change, advancing health.* Washington, DC: National Academies Press. Retrieved from http://www.thefutureofnursing.org/IOM-Report

Lloyd Sealy Library. (2015). Evaluating information sources. Retrieved from http://guides.lib.jjay.cuny.edu/evaluatingsources

Rosseter, R. J. (2015). Fact sheet: The impact of education on nursing practice. American Association of Colleges of Nursing. Retrieved from www.aacn.nche.edu/media-relations/Edimpact.pdf

Smith, J. (2003). Exploring the values of continuing education mandates. Retrieved from http://www.ncsbn.org/CEStudy.pdf

Xu, E. (2013). RN vs. BSN: What you should know. Rasmussen College. Retrieved from http://www.rasmussen.edu/degrees/nursing/blog/rn-vs-bsn-what-you-should-know

INDEX

A

AAACN (American Academy of Ambulatory Care Nursing), 146

AACN (American Association of Colleges of Nursing), 159–160, 168

AACN (American Association of Critical-Care Nurses), 168

accountability, 93, 98

ADN (associate degree in nursing)
  characteristics, 7, 158–159
  history, 6

advance directive, 66

advance medical care directive, 66

advanced degrees. *See* nursing advanced degrees

advocate, 66

ambulatory care
  American Academy of Ambulatory Care Nursing (AAACN), 146
  RN roles in, 146

American Association for Long Term Care Nursing, 151

American Association of Colleges of Nursing (AACN), 159–160, 168

L

RN workforce statistics, 140,
142–143, 160
school nursing
National Association of
School Nurses (NASN),
153
RN roles in, 153
professional roles. *See* roles of
registered nurses
professionalism, 105–106
public health
Association of Public Health
Nurses, 148
RN roles in, 147
U.S. public health system
(PHS), 147–148
websites related to, 148

R

reality shock, 112
registered nurses. *See* roles of
registered nurses
REM sleep, 30
residency programs
and *The Future of Nursing*
report, 16
how to find, 17
RN-to-BSN degrees, 17–19
roles of licensed practical nurses/
licensed vocational nurses. *See
also* roles of registered nurses
employment opportunities,
52
responsibilities of, 52–53
scope of practice, 52, 54

roles of registered nurses. *See
also* roles of licensed practical nurses/licensed vocational
nurses
in ambulatory care nursing,
146
ANA Standards of Nursing
Practice and Professional
Performance, 44–45
in home health nursing,
148–149
in hospice nursing, 150
leadership roles, 50–51
in long-term care nursing,
150–153
nursing as profession, 40–42
professional involvement, 43
professional practice, 42
clinical autonomy, 43–44
control over practice,
43–44
in public health nursing,
147–148
in school nursing, 153
scope of practice, 36, 44
specialty standards of practice, 46
as team member, 52–53

S

SBAR-R communication (Situation, Background, Assessment,
Recommendation, Read back
and Verify), 100

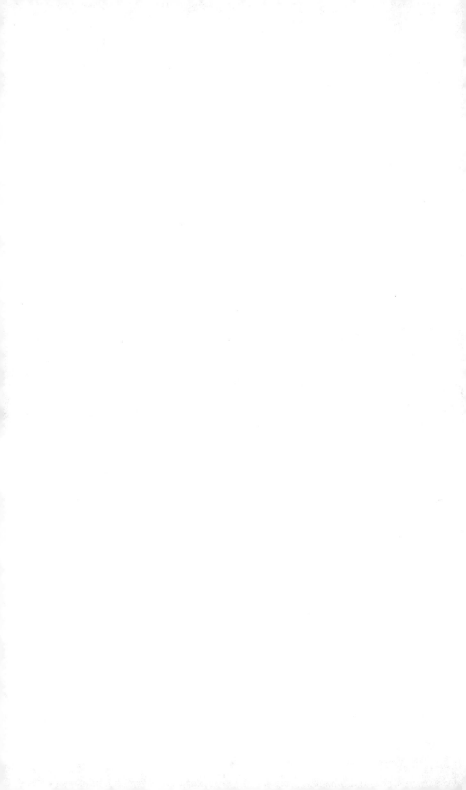

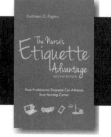
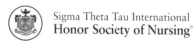
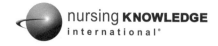

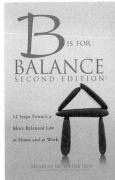
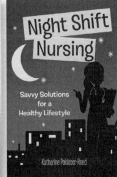
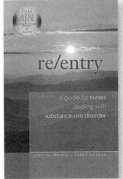
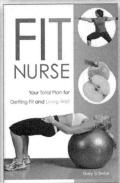

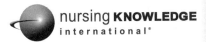

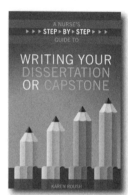
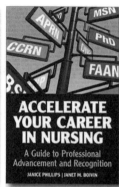
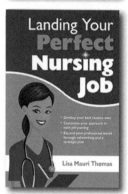
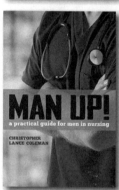

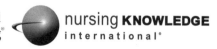